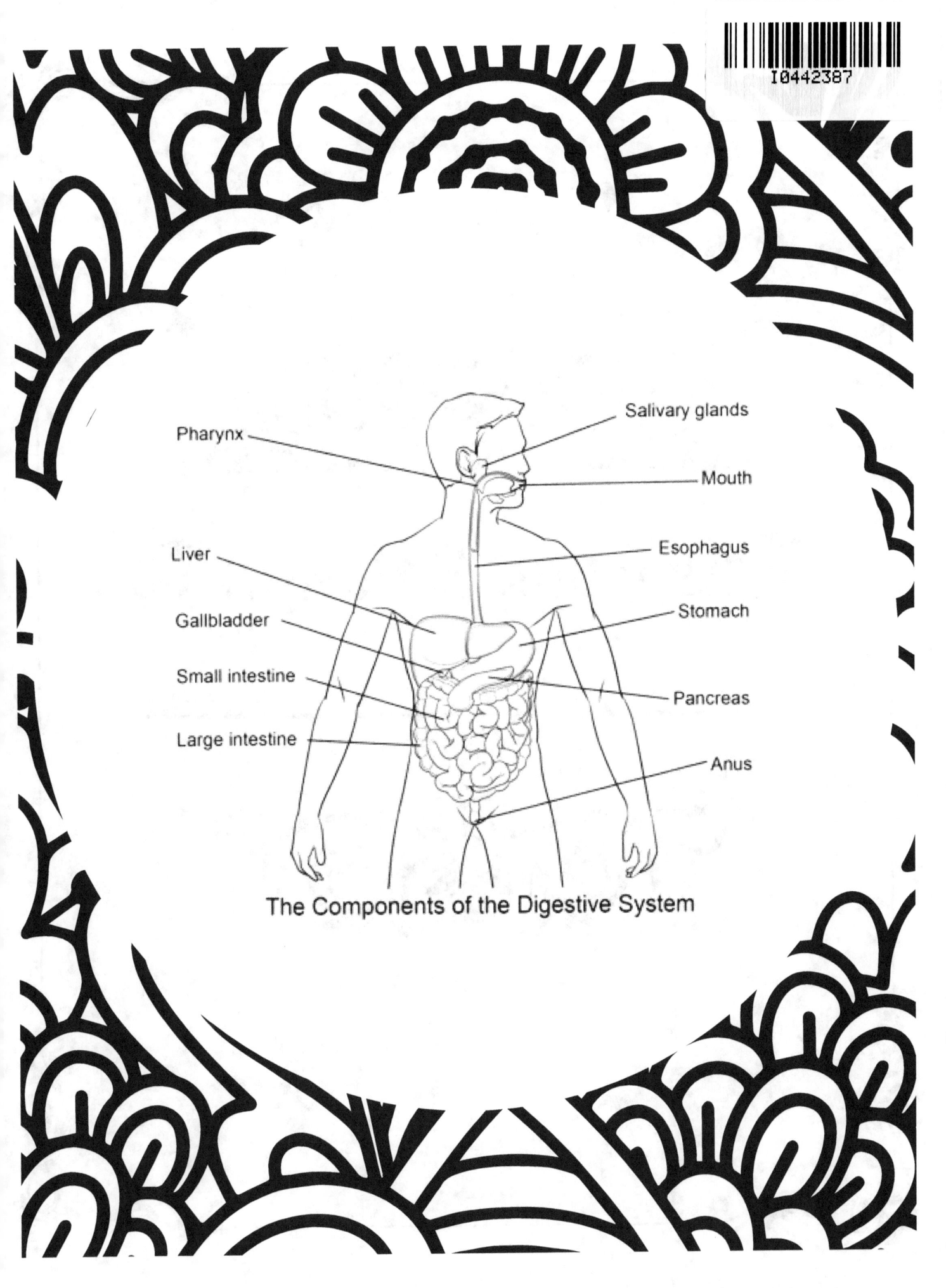

The Components of the Digestive System

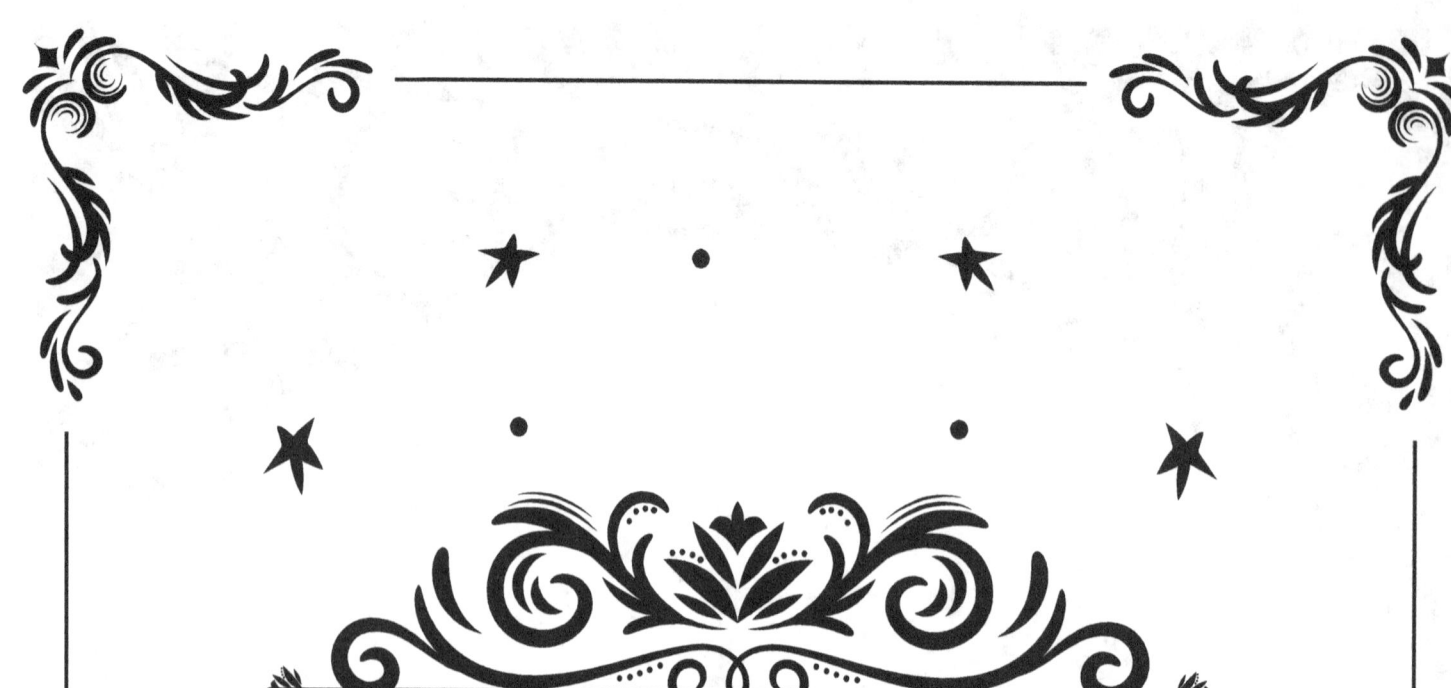

This Book Belongs To

_____

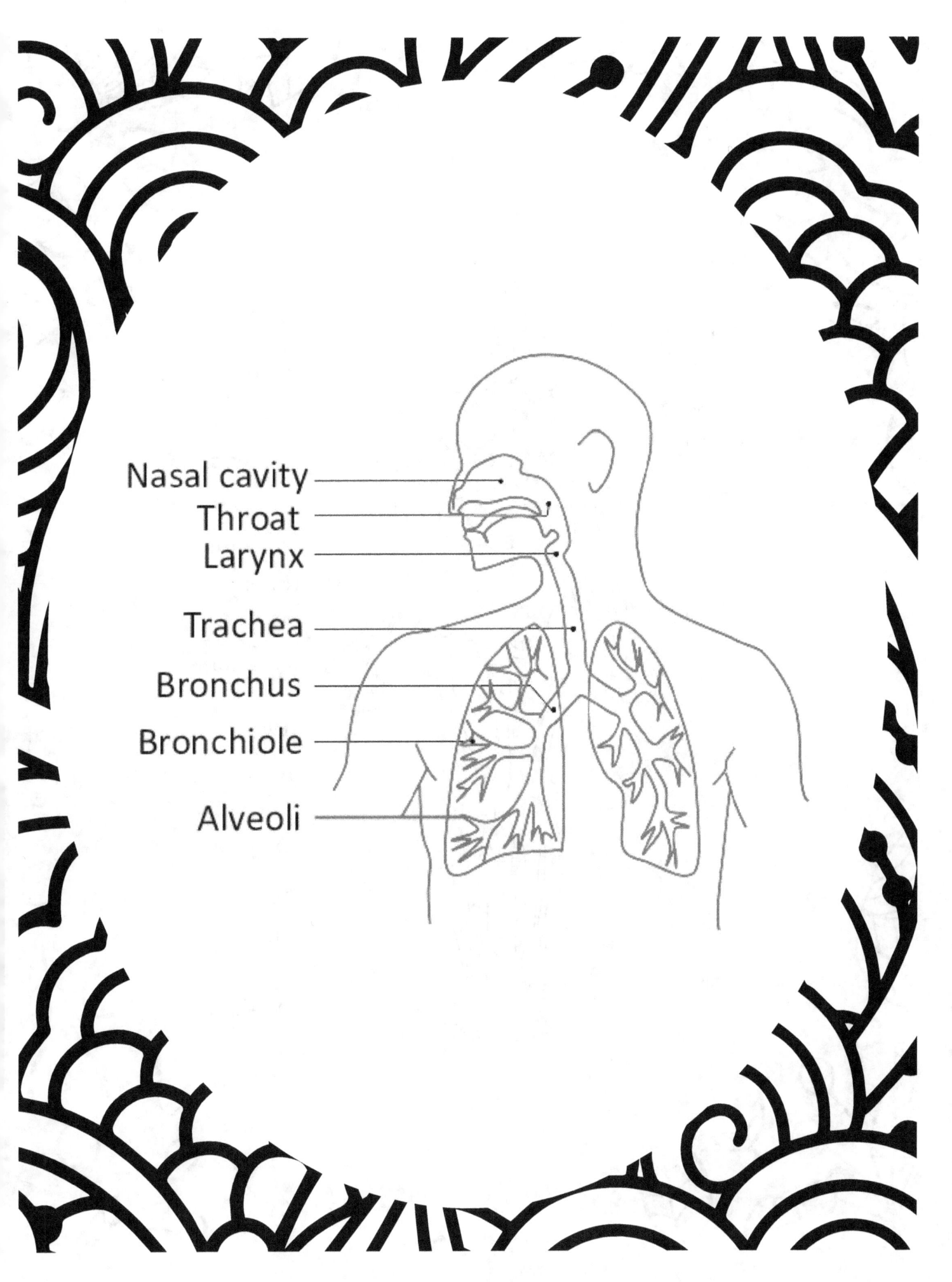

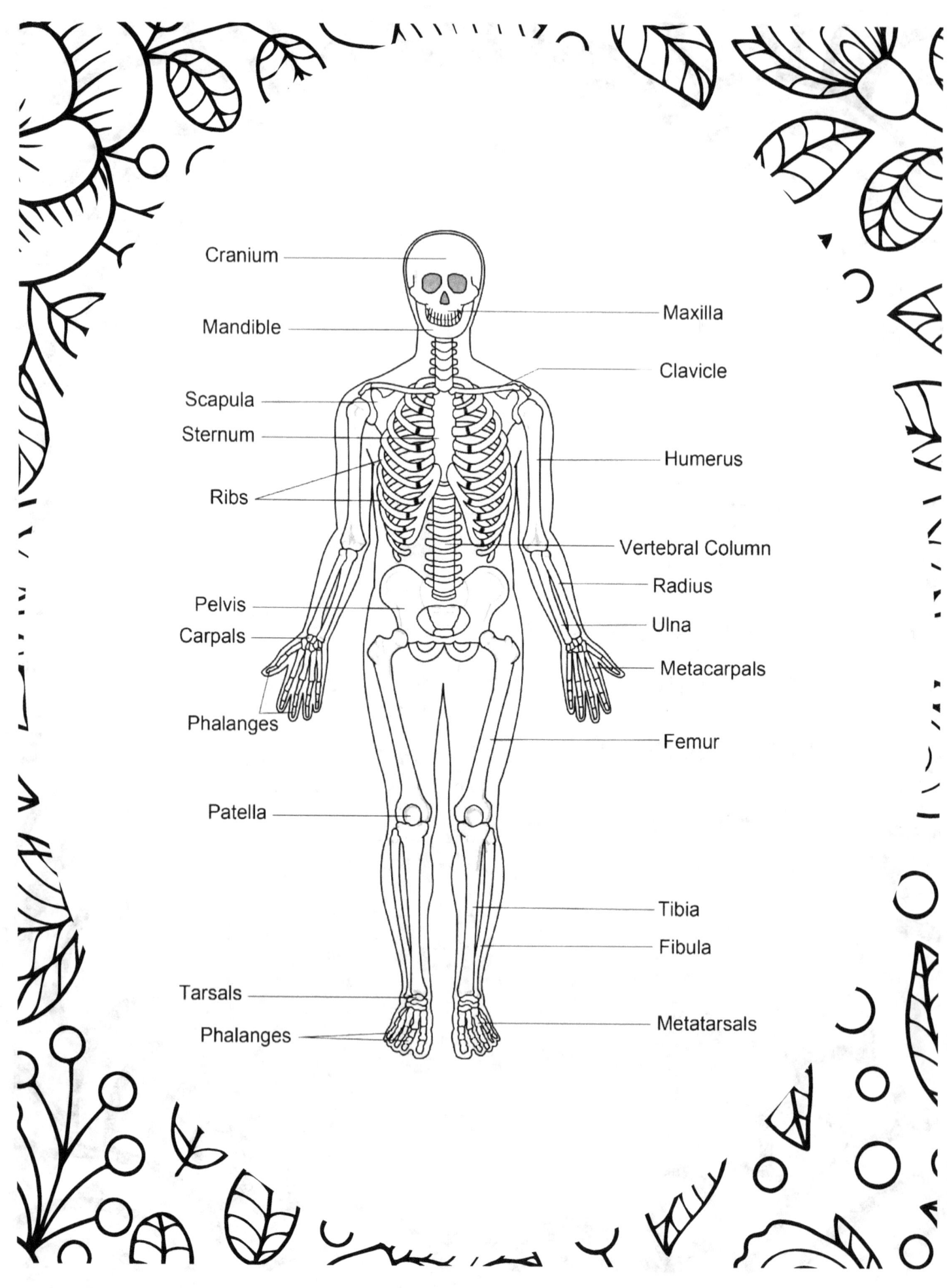

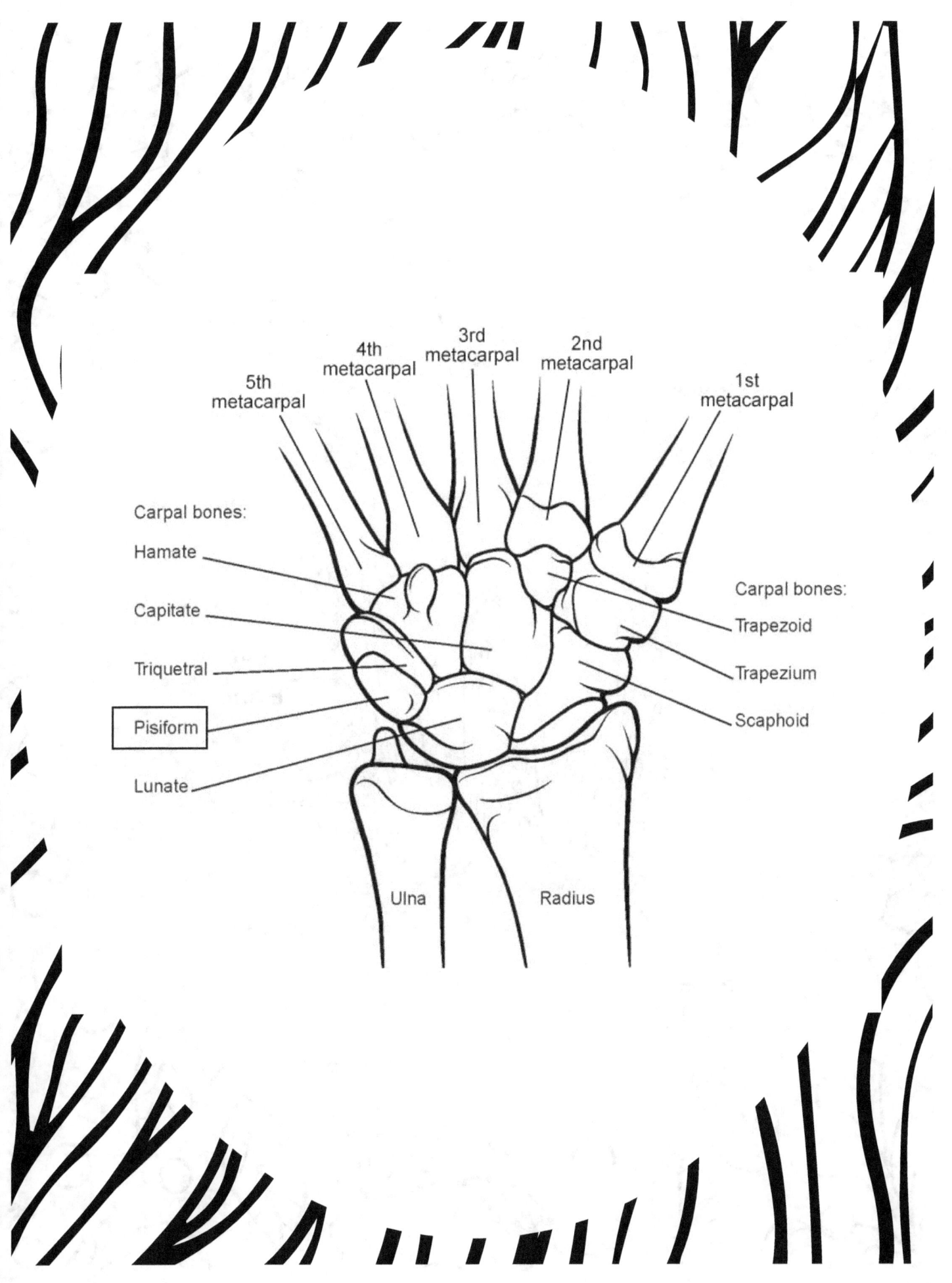

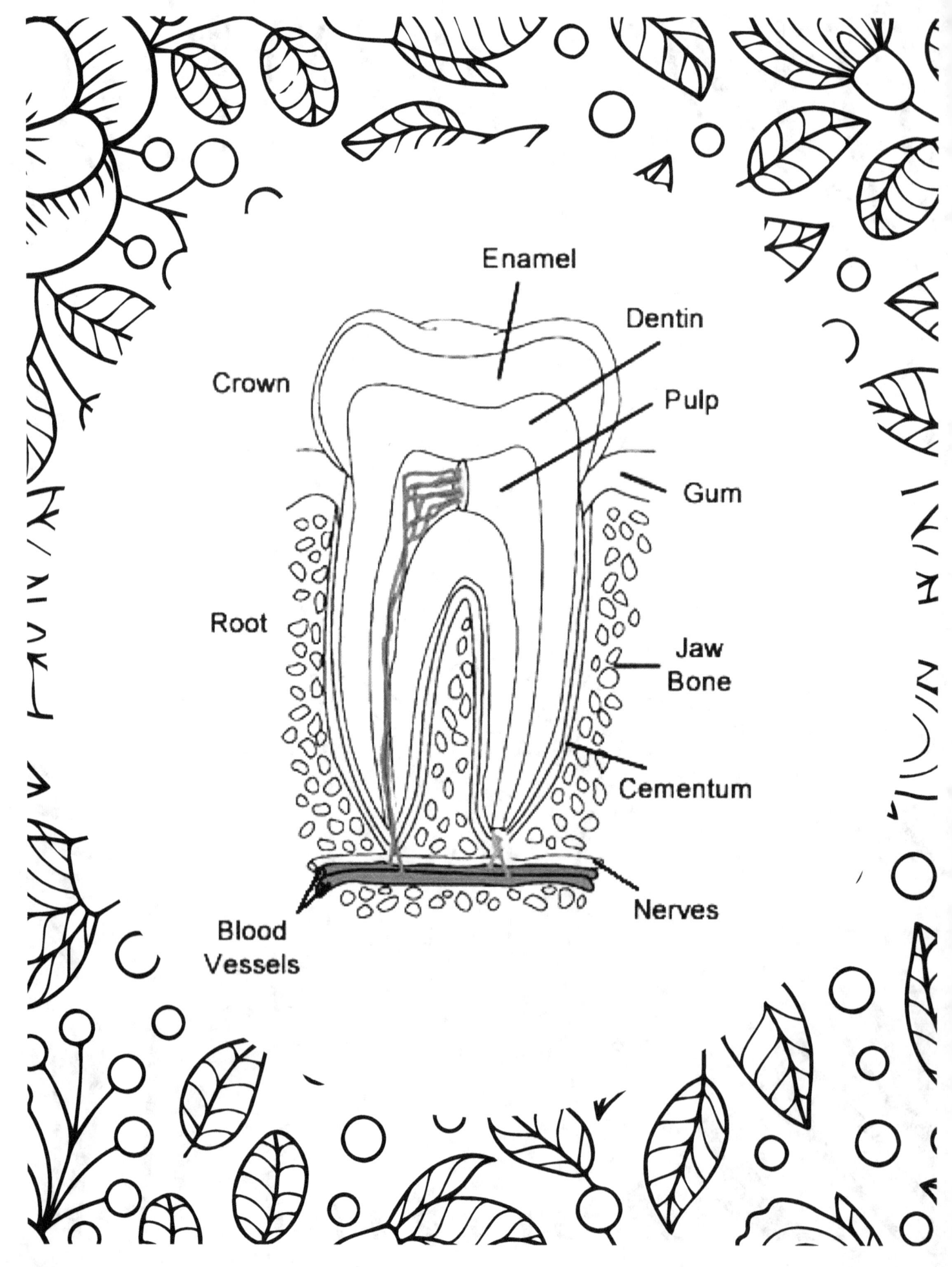

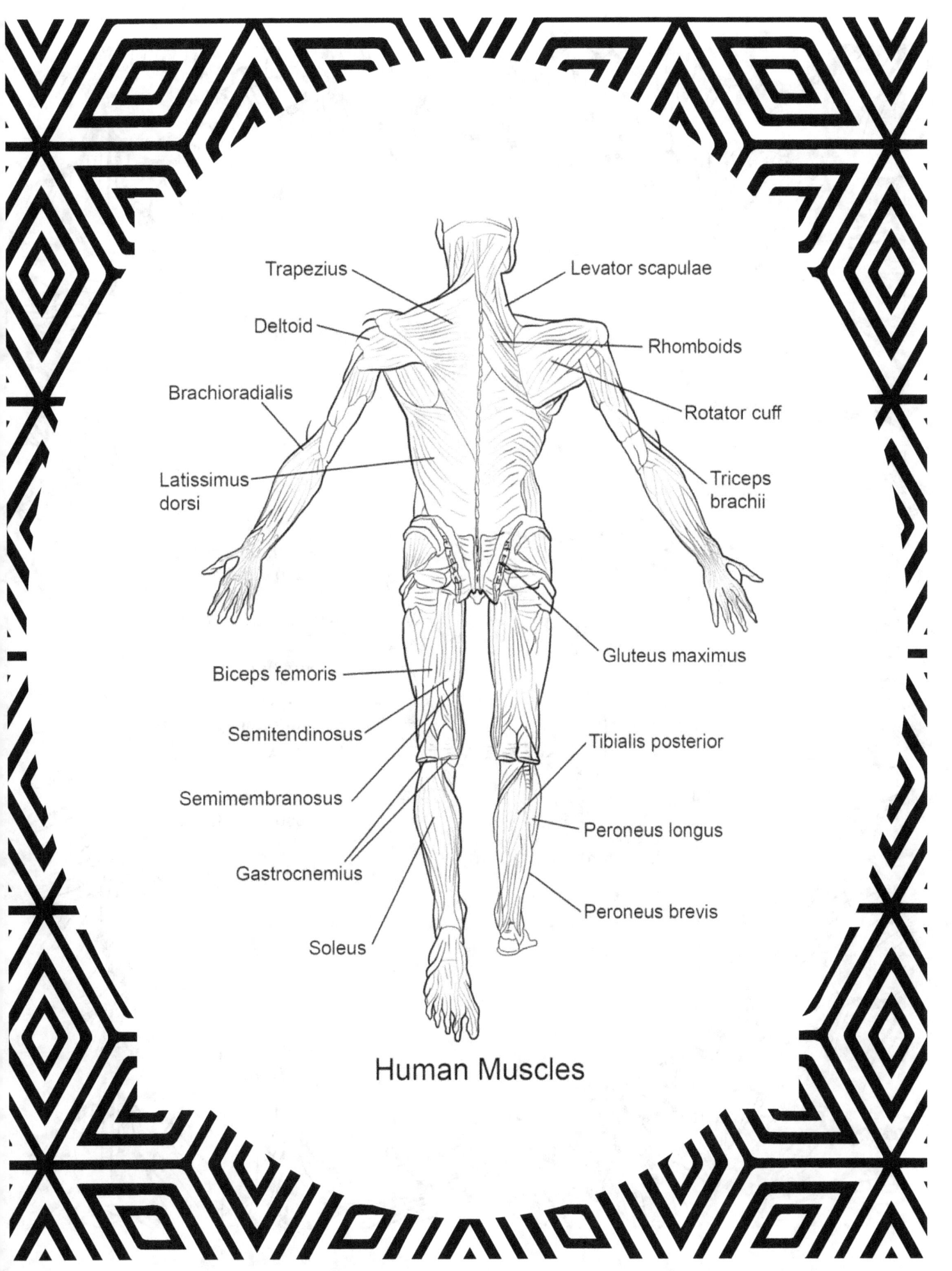

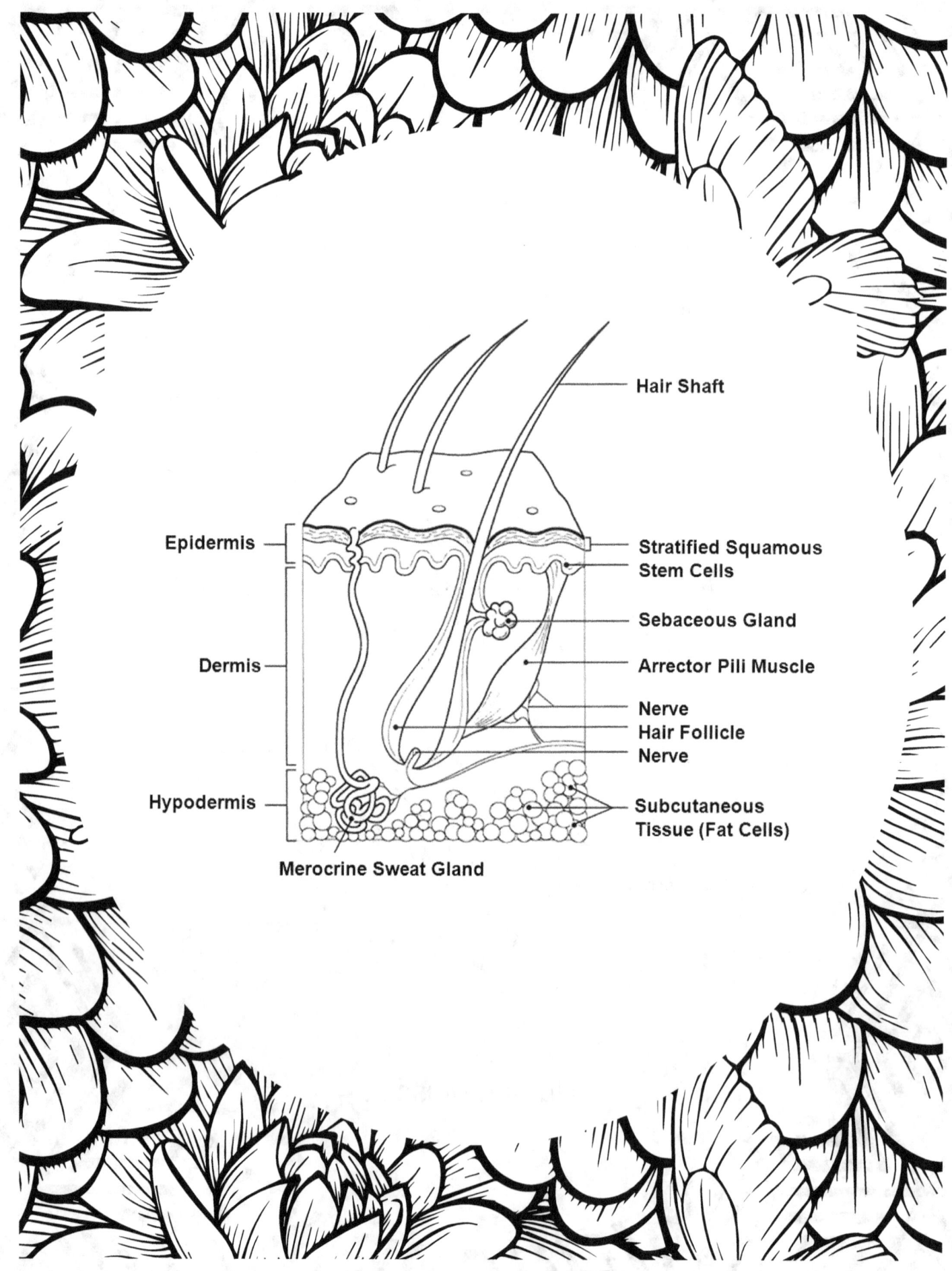

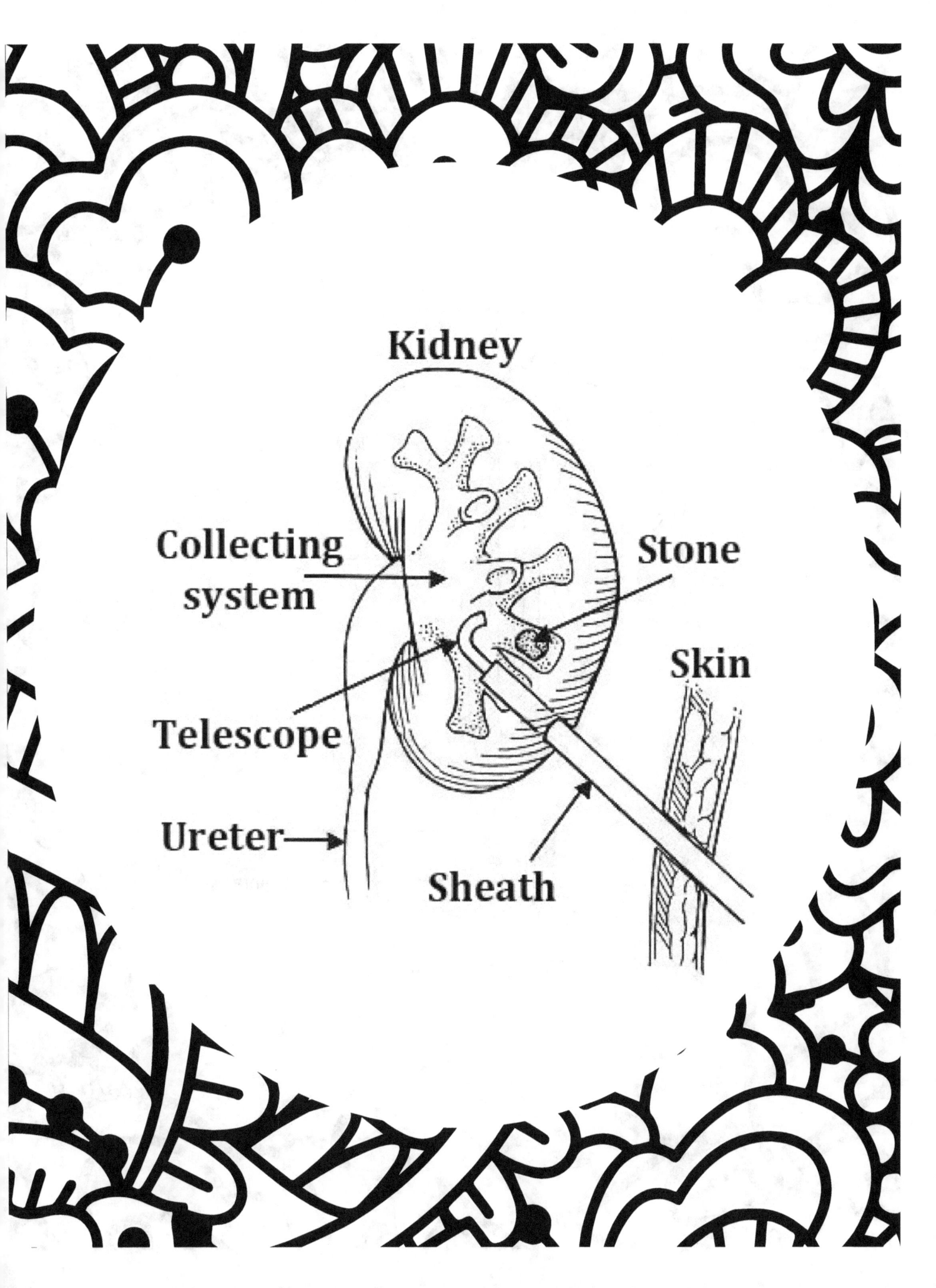

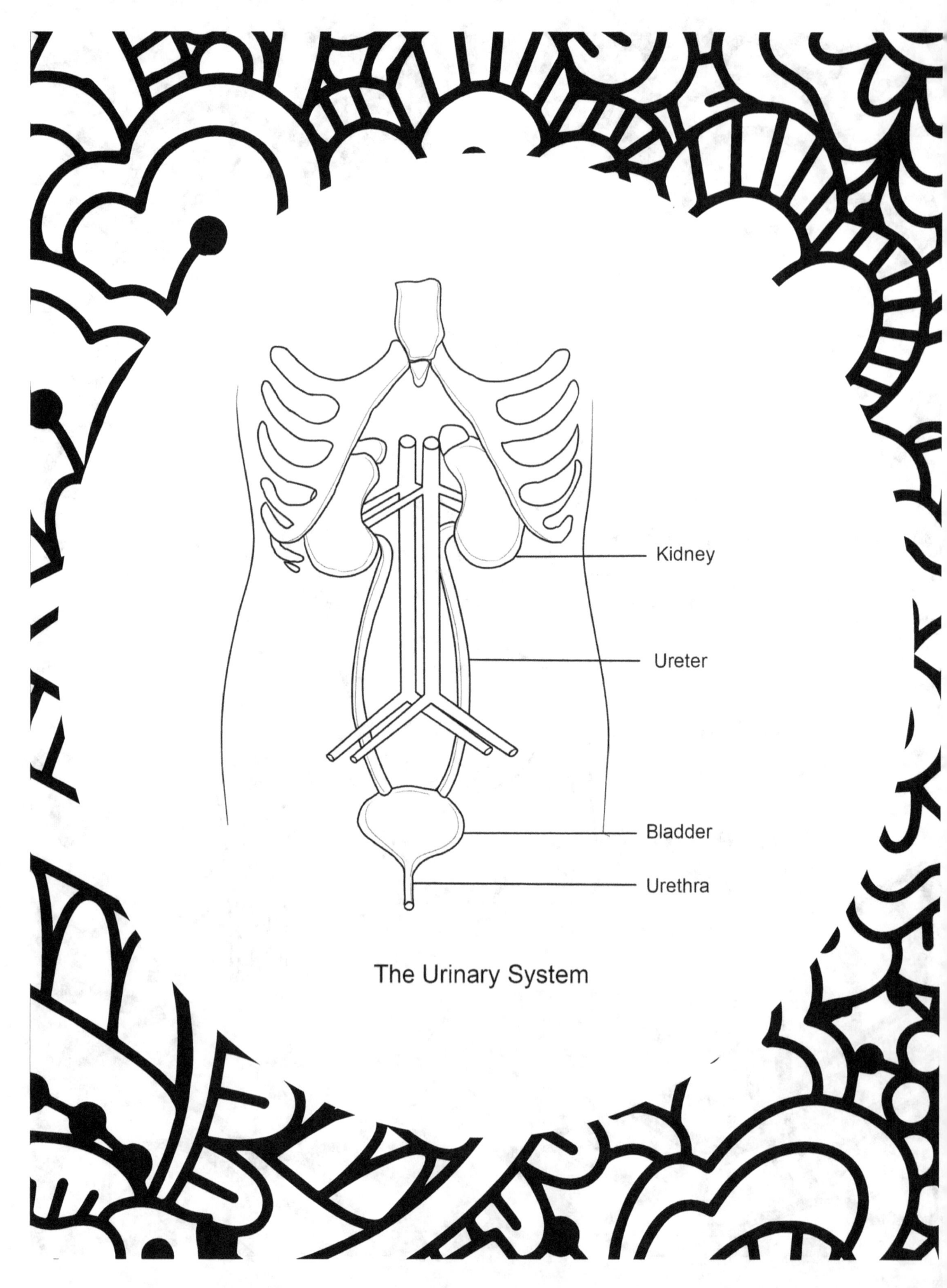

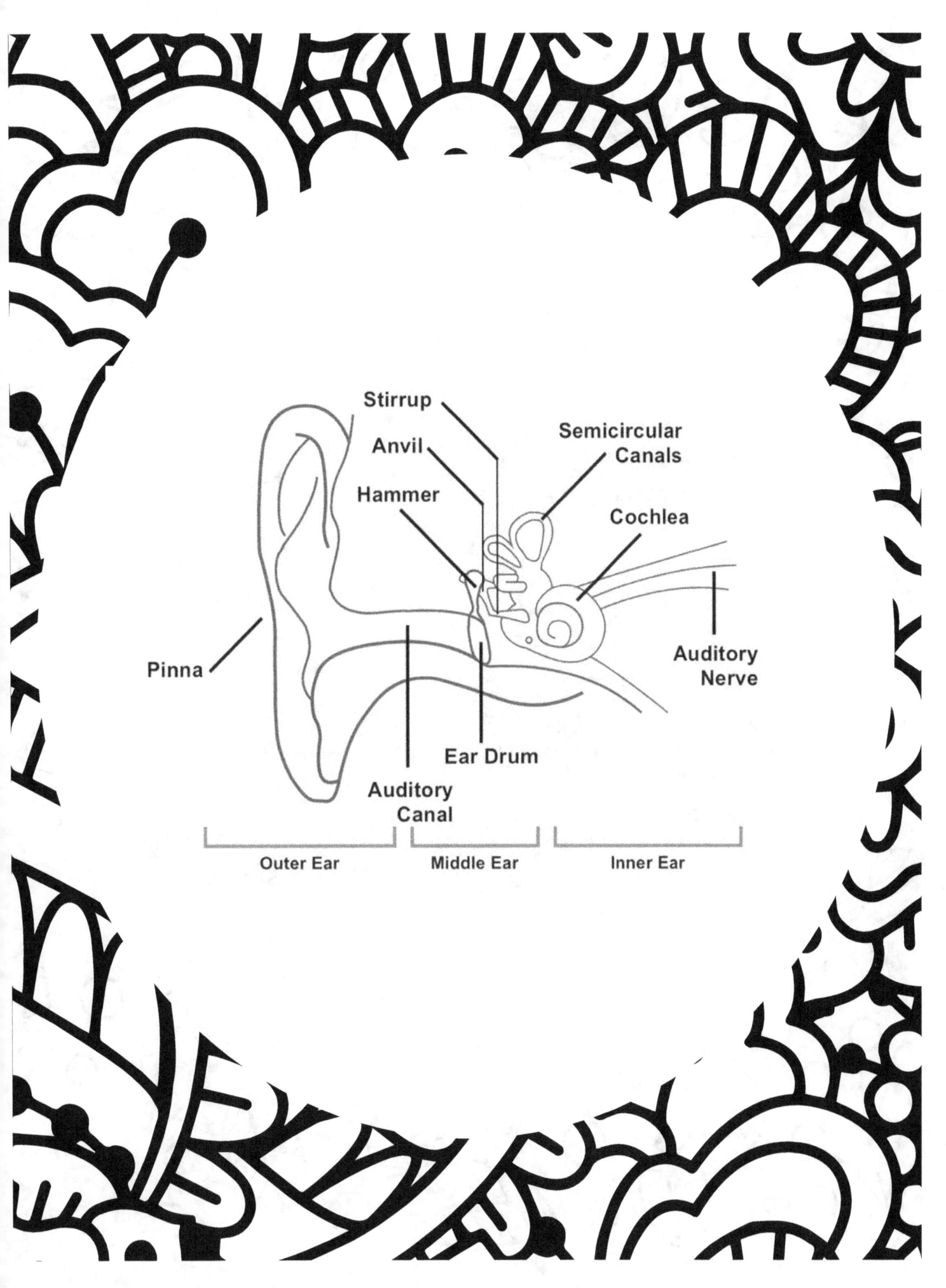

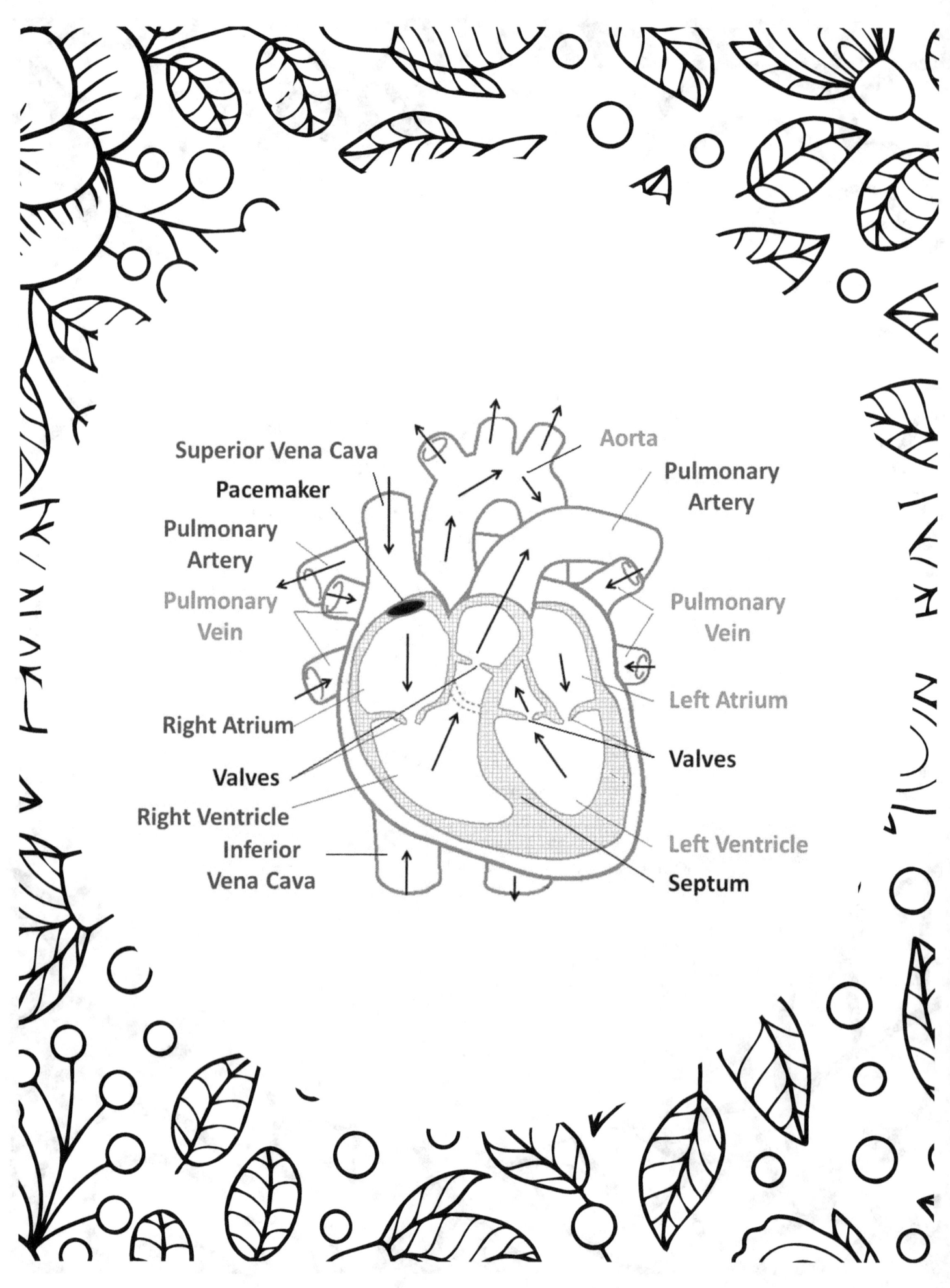

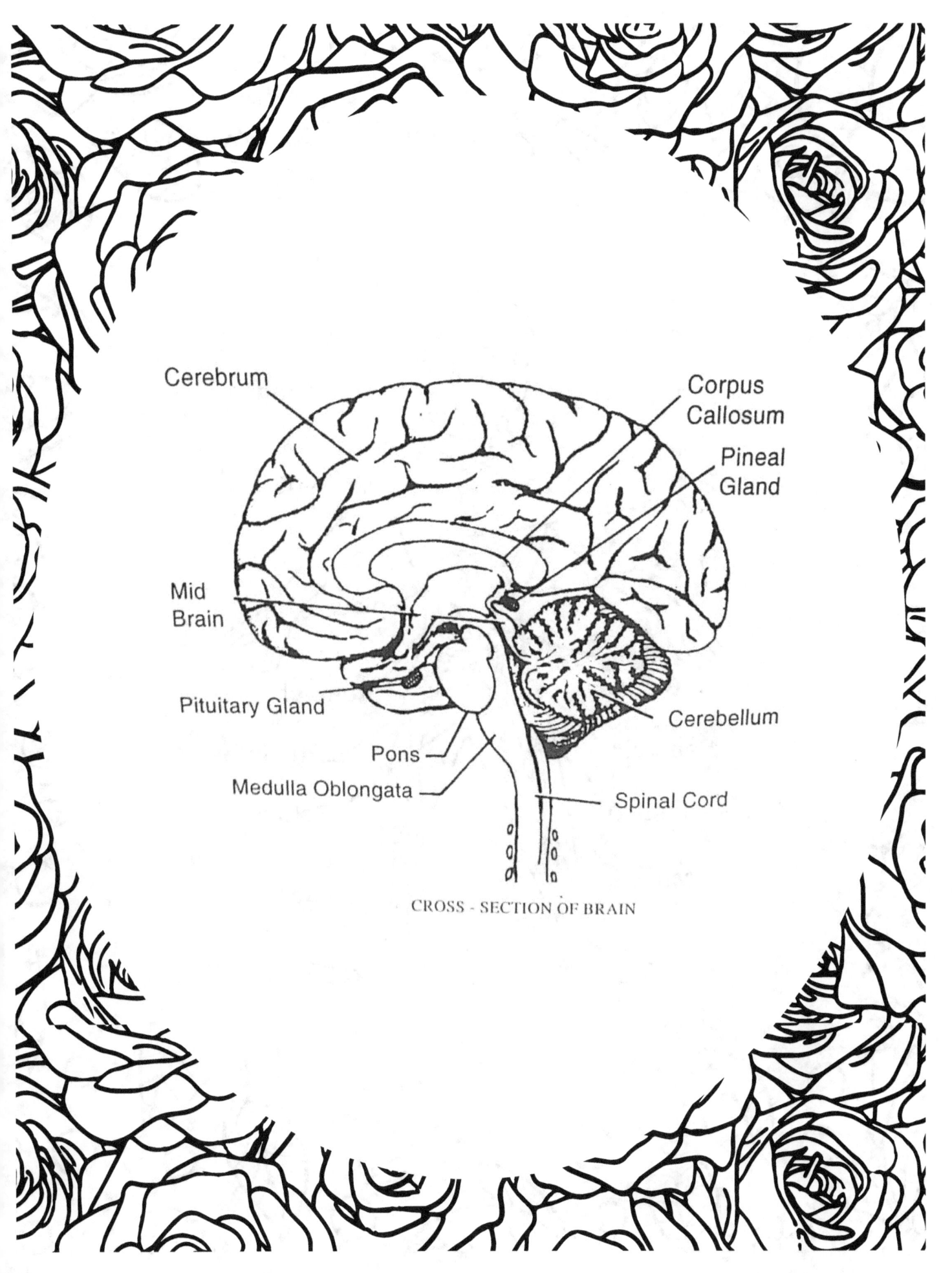

CROSS - SECTION OF BRAIN

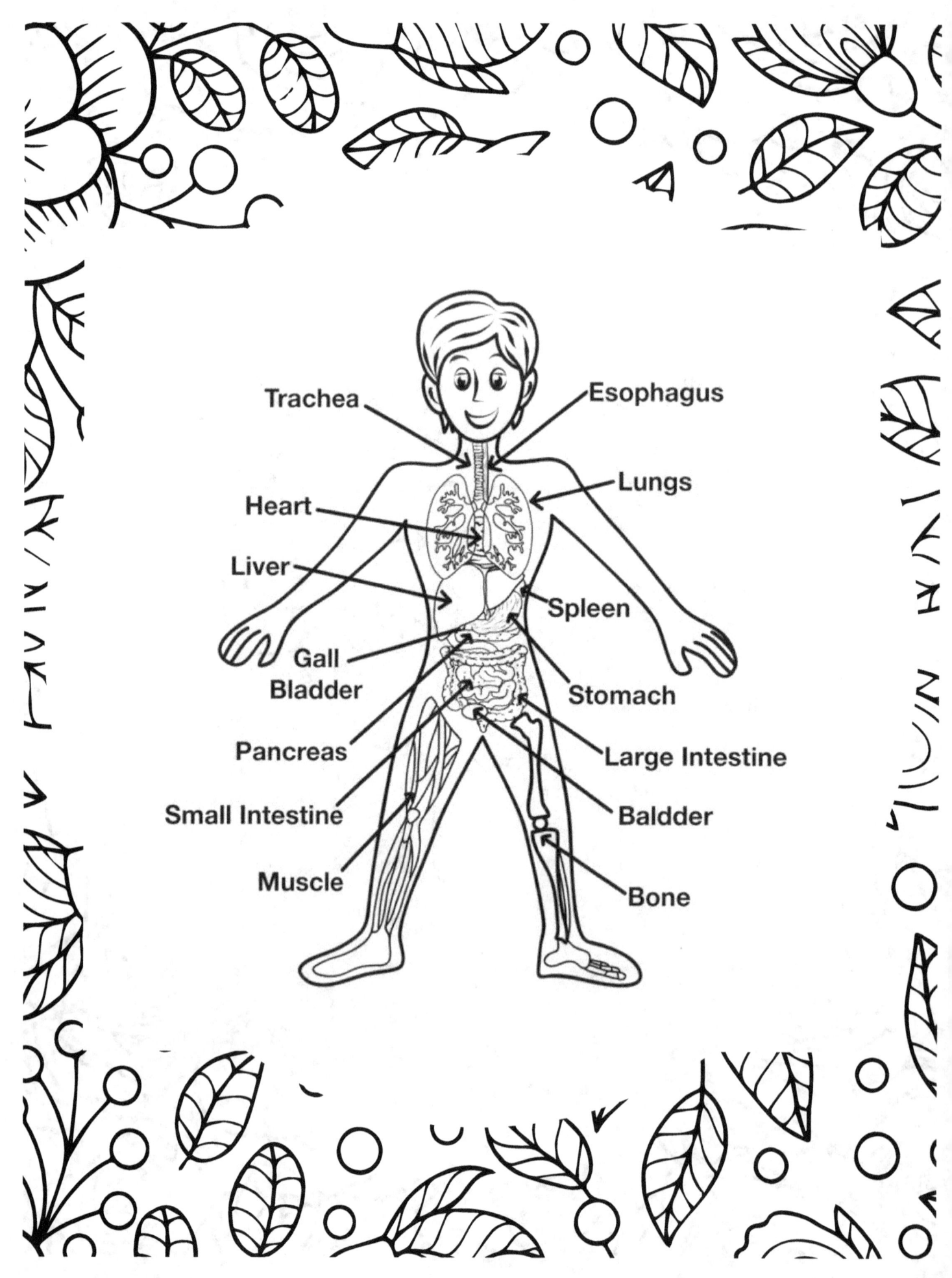

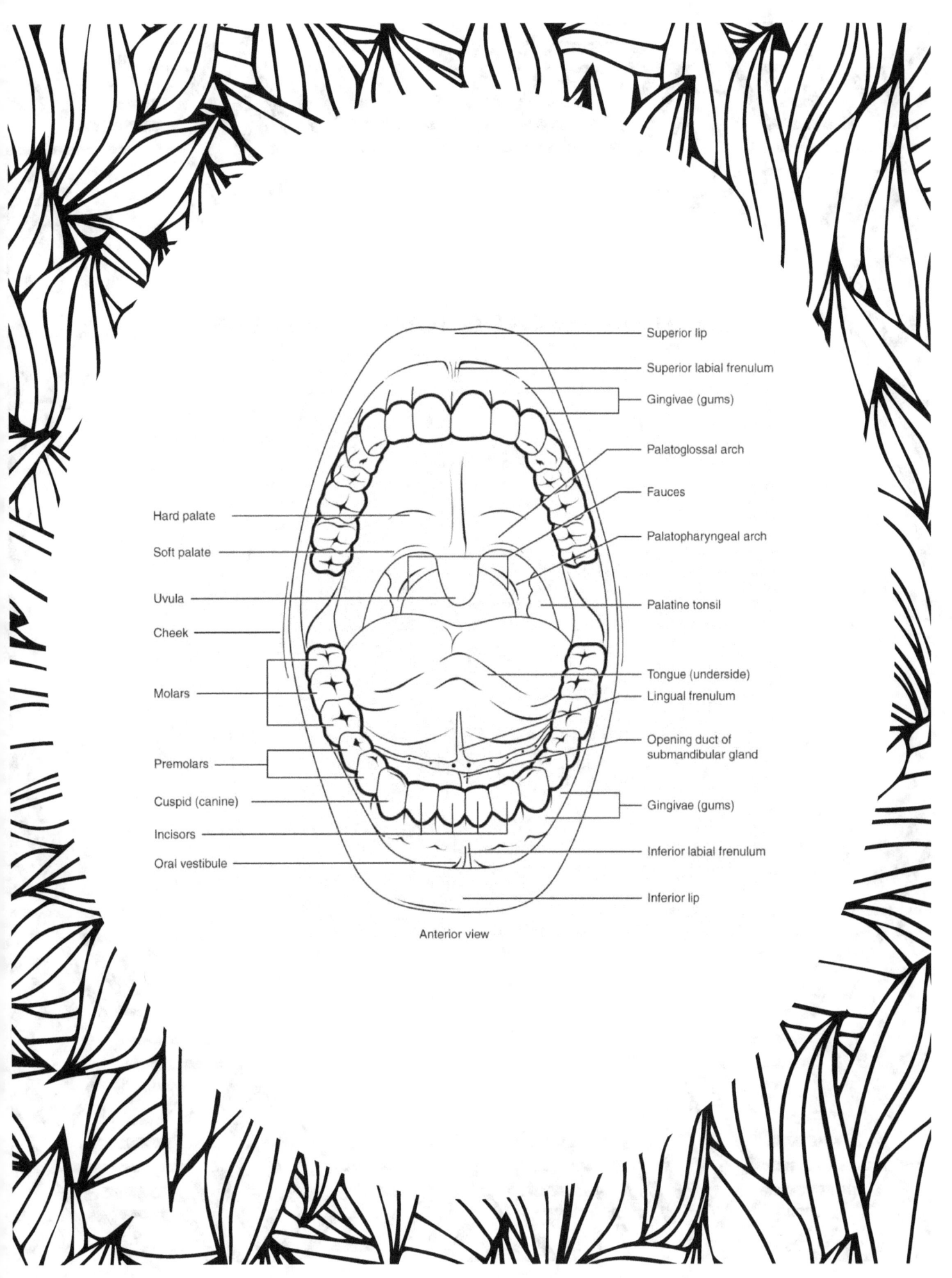

Anterior view

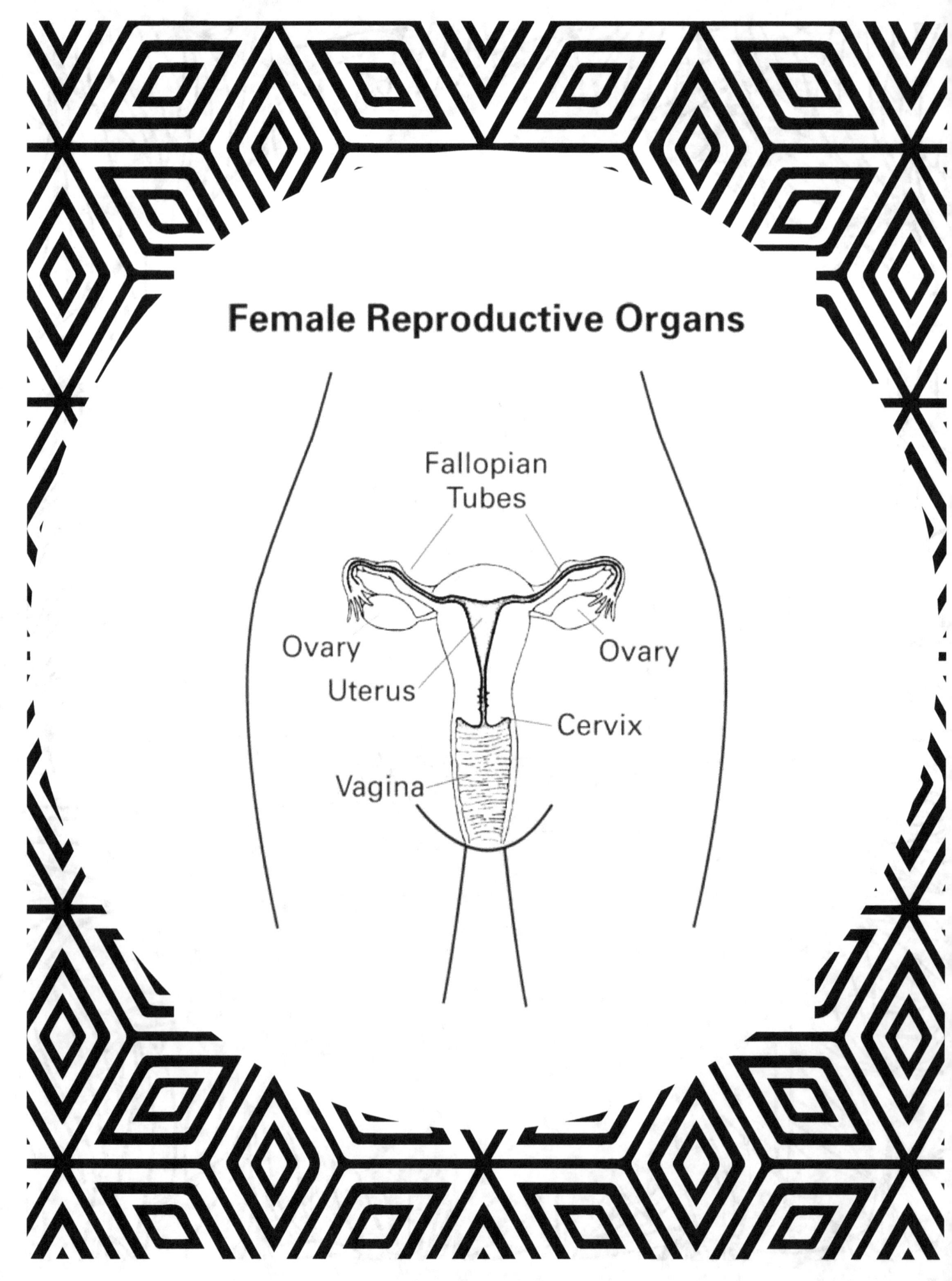

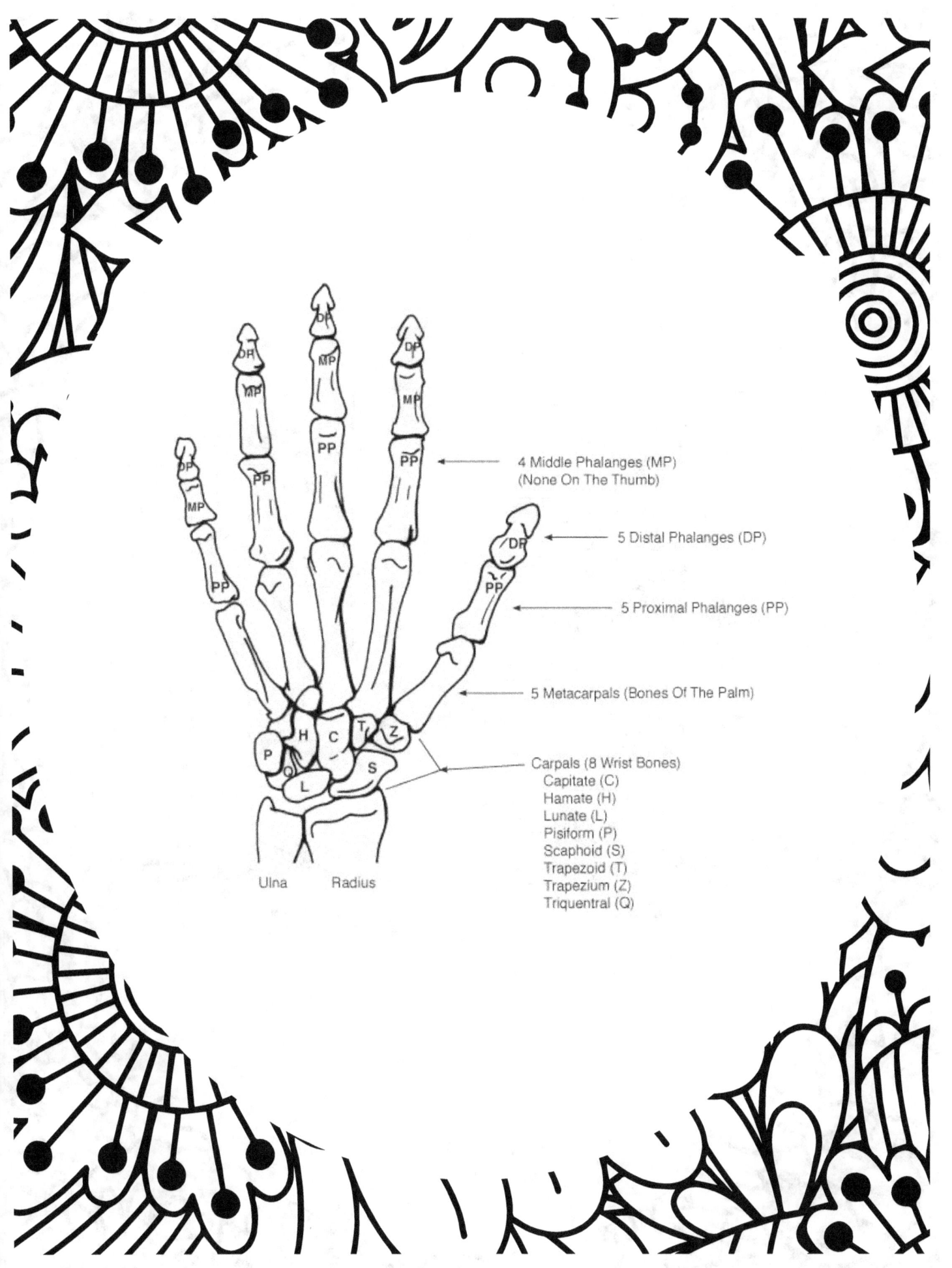

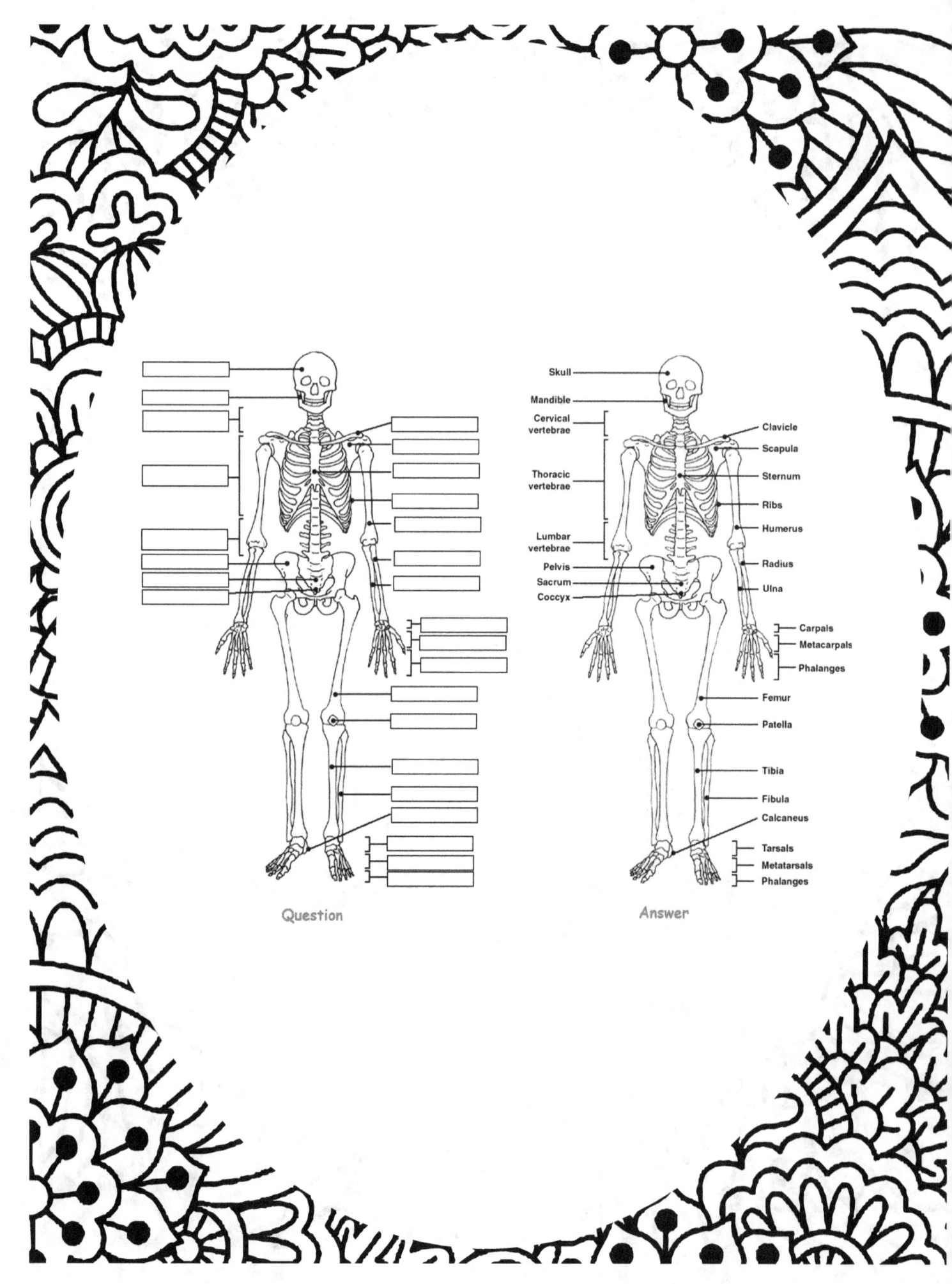

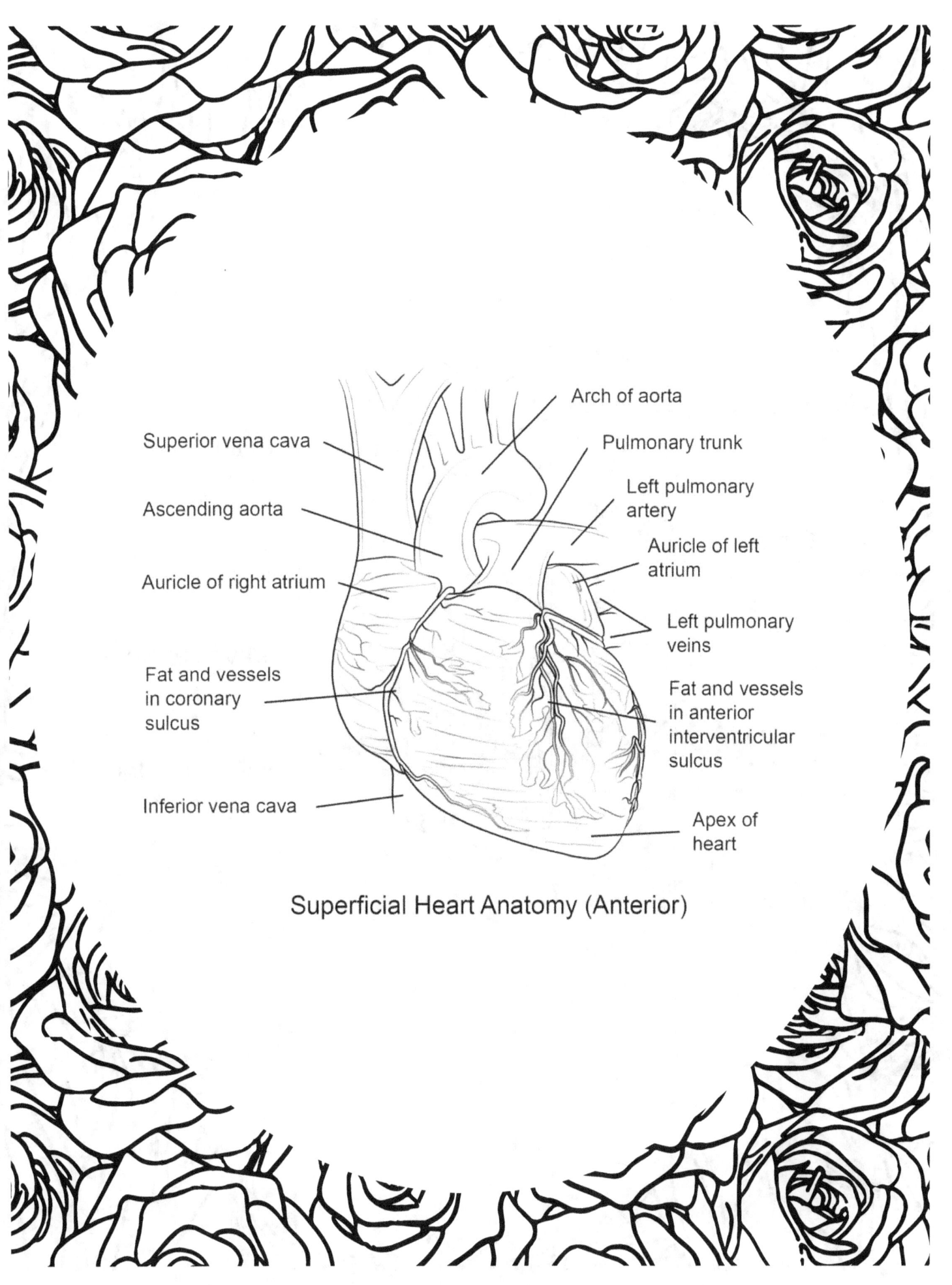

Superficial Heart Anatomy (Anterior)

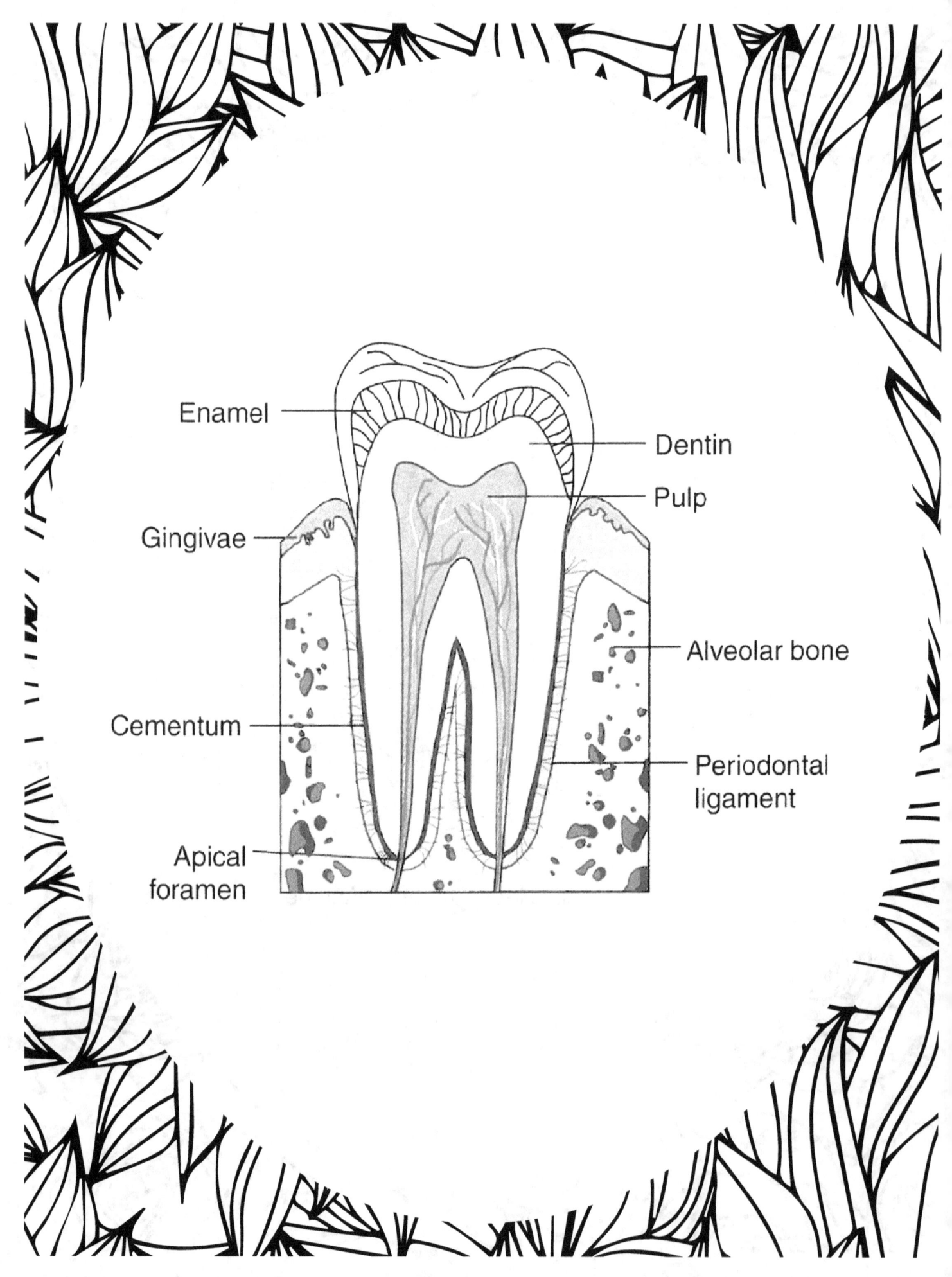

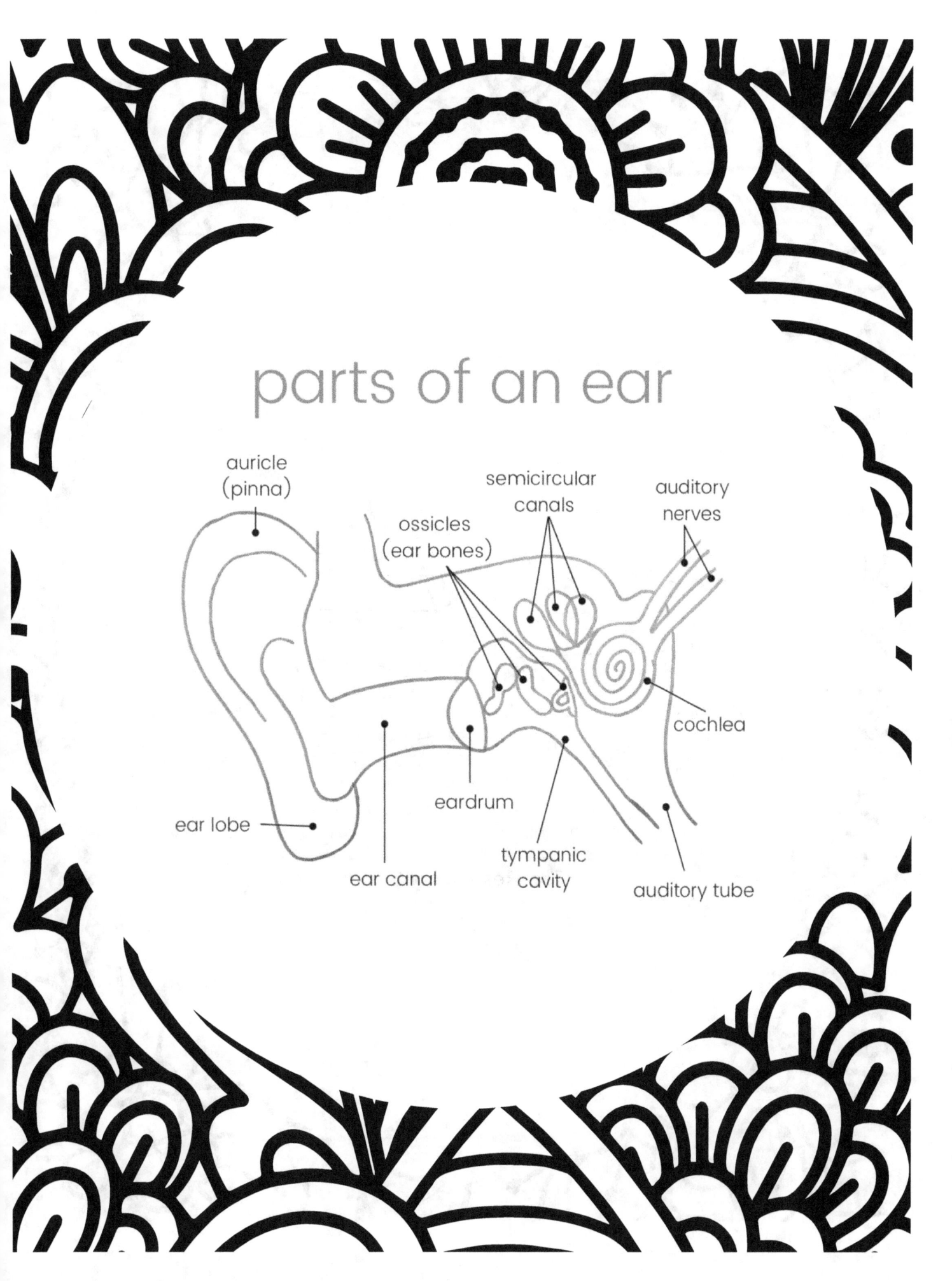

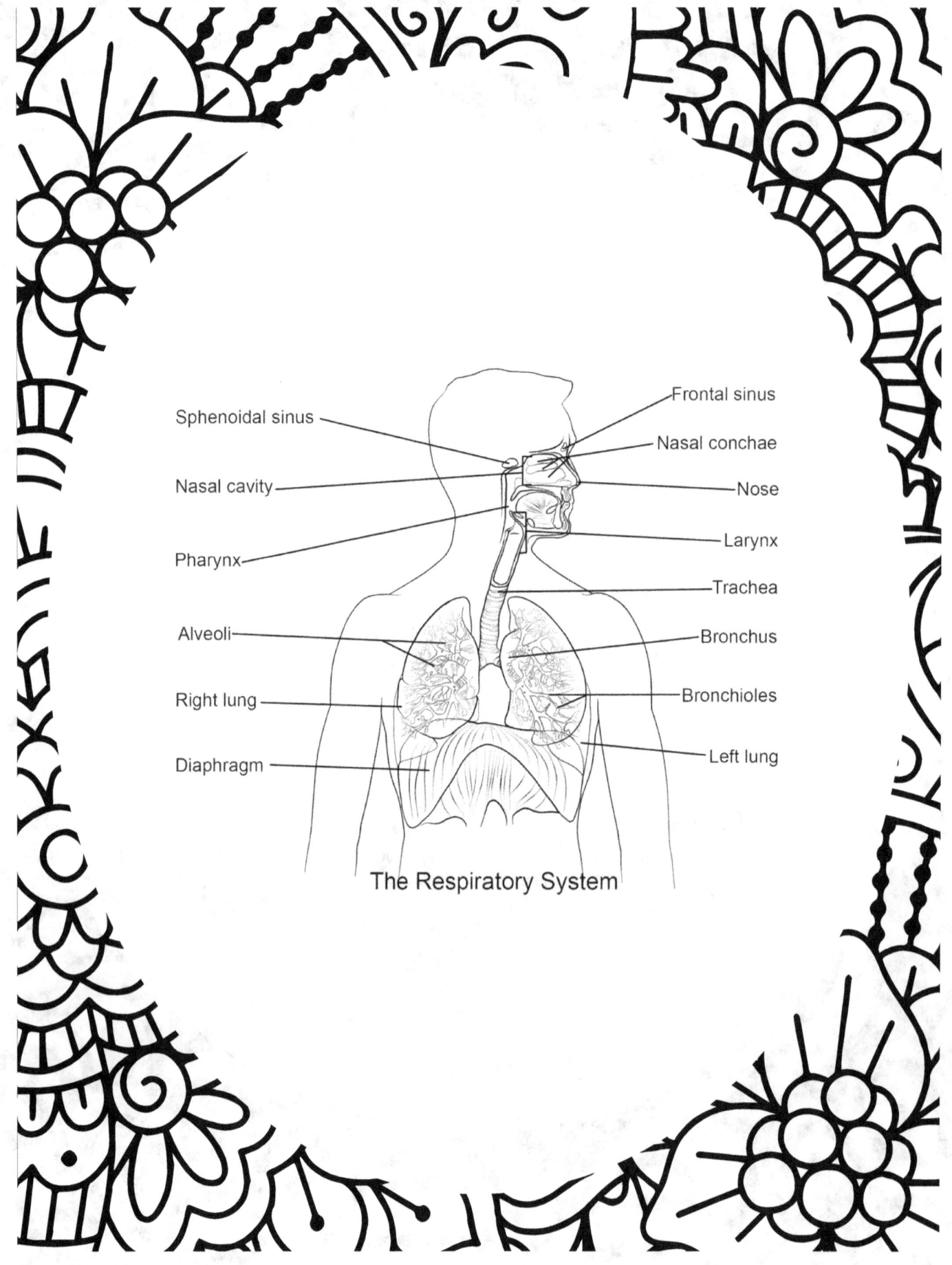

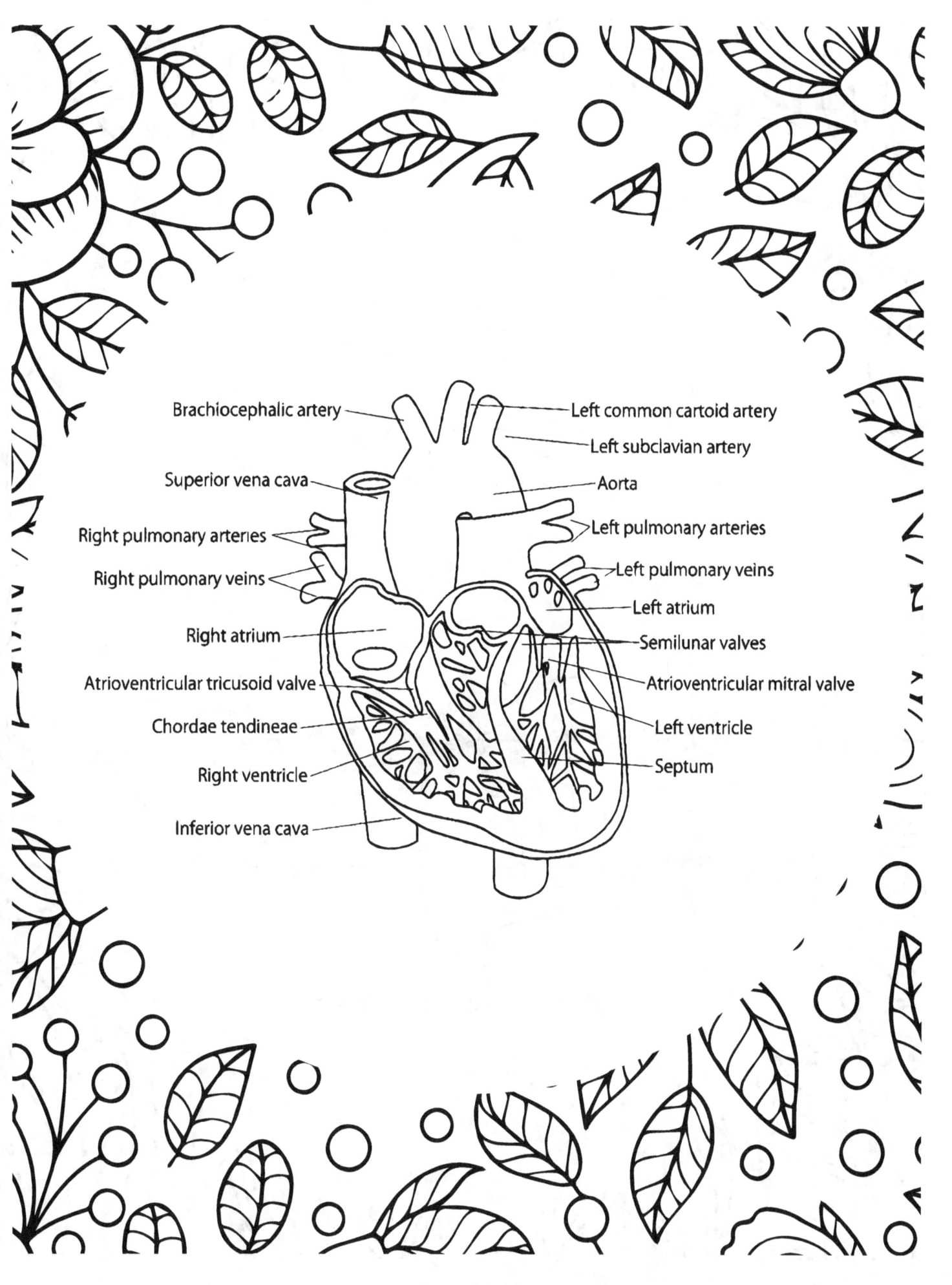

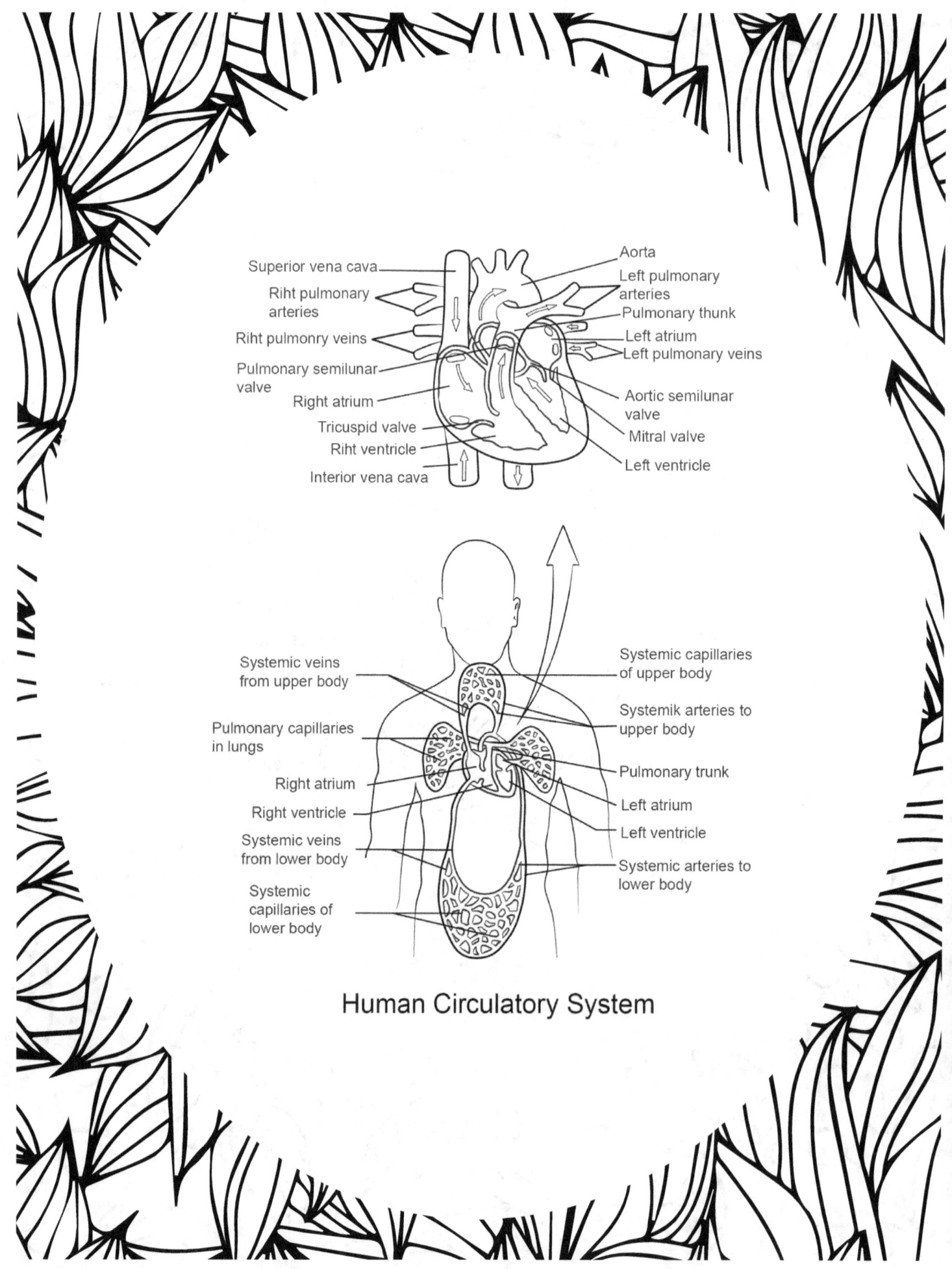

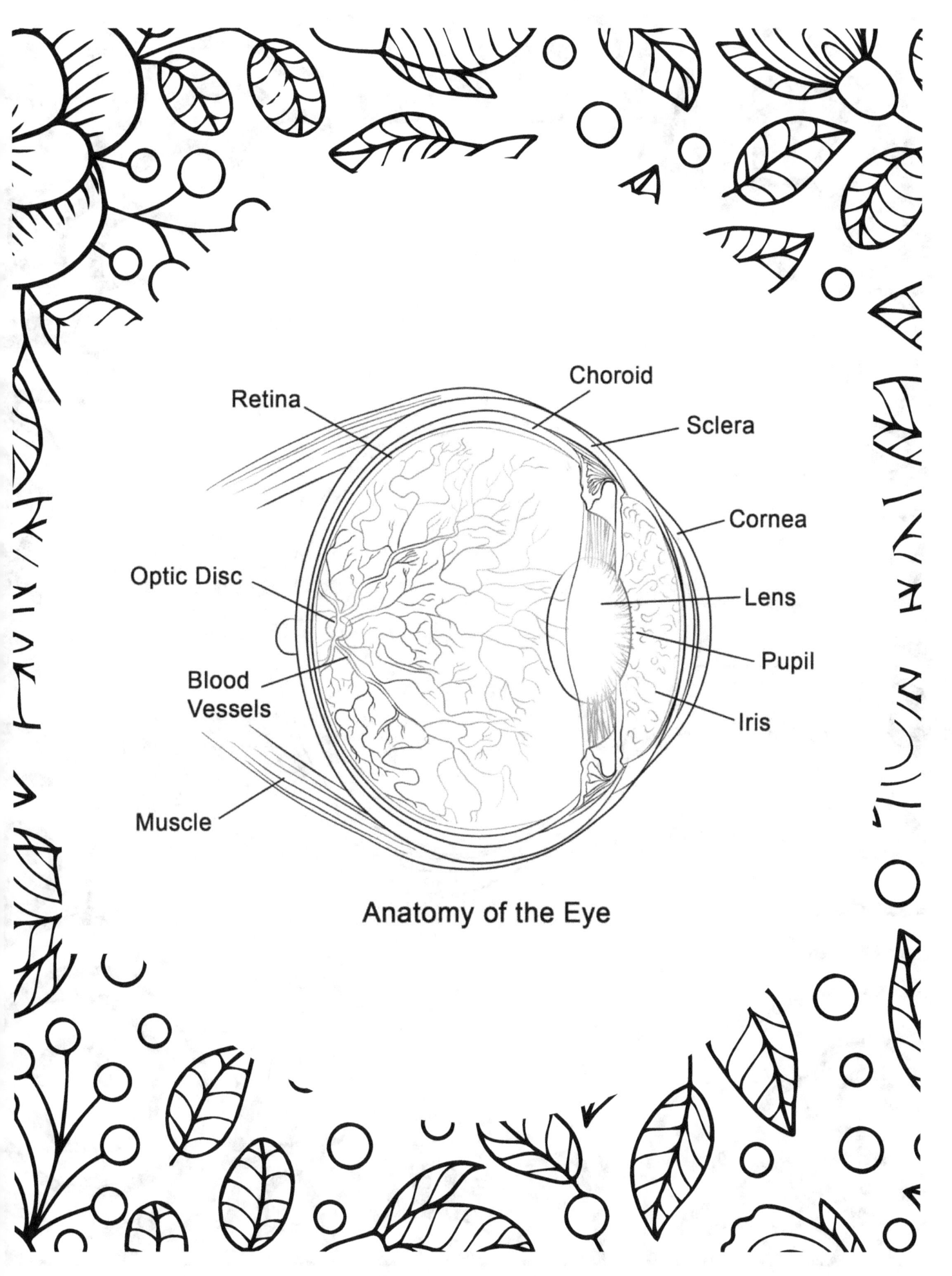

Anatomy of the Eye

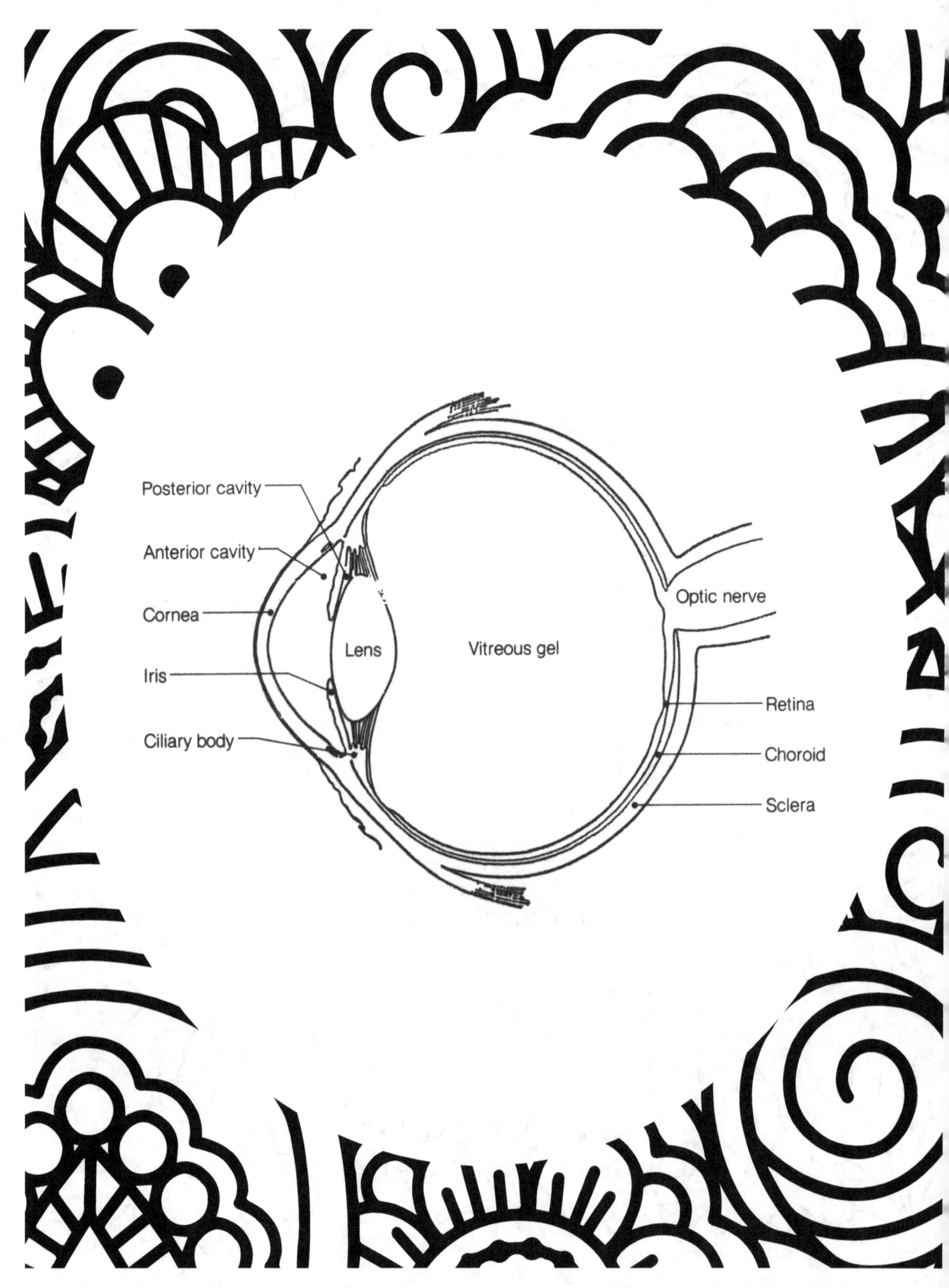

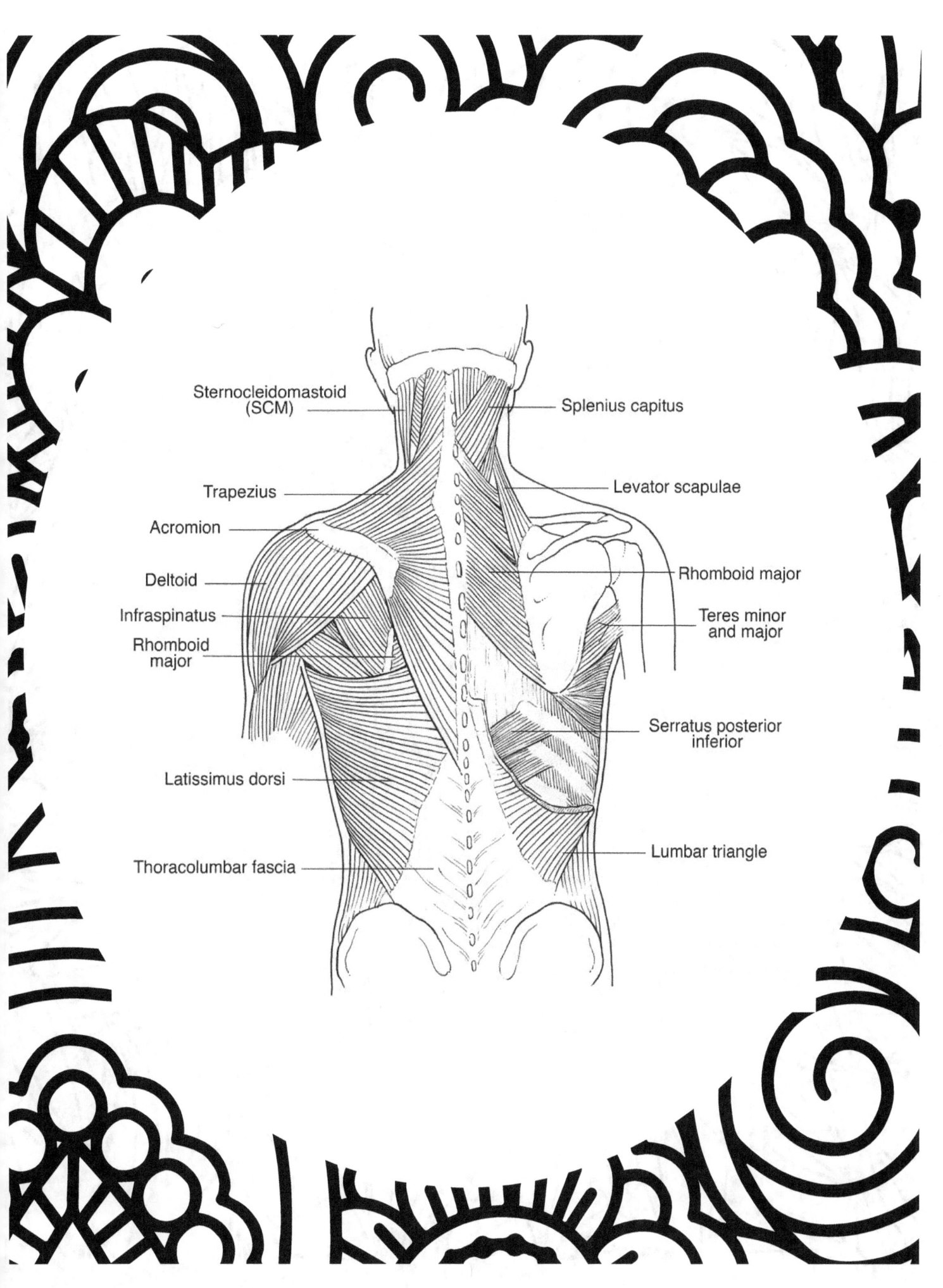

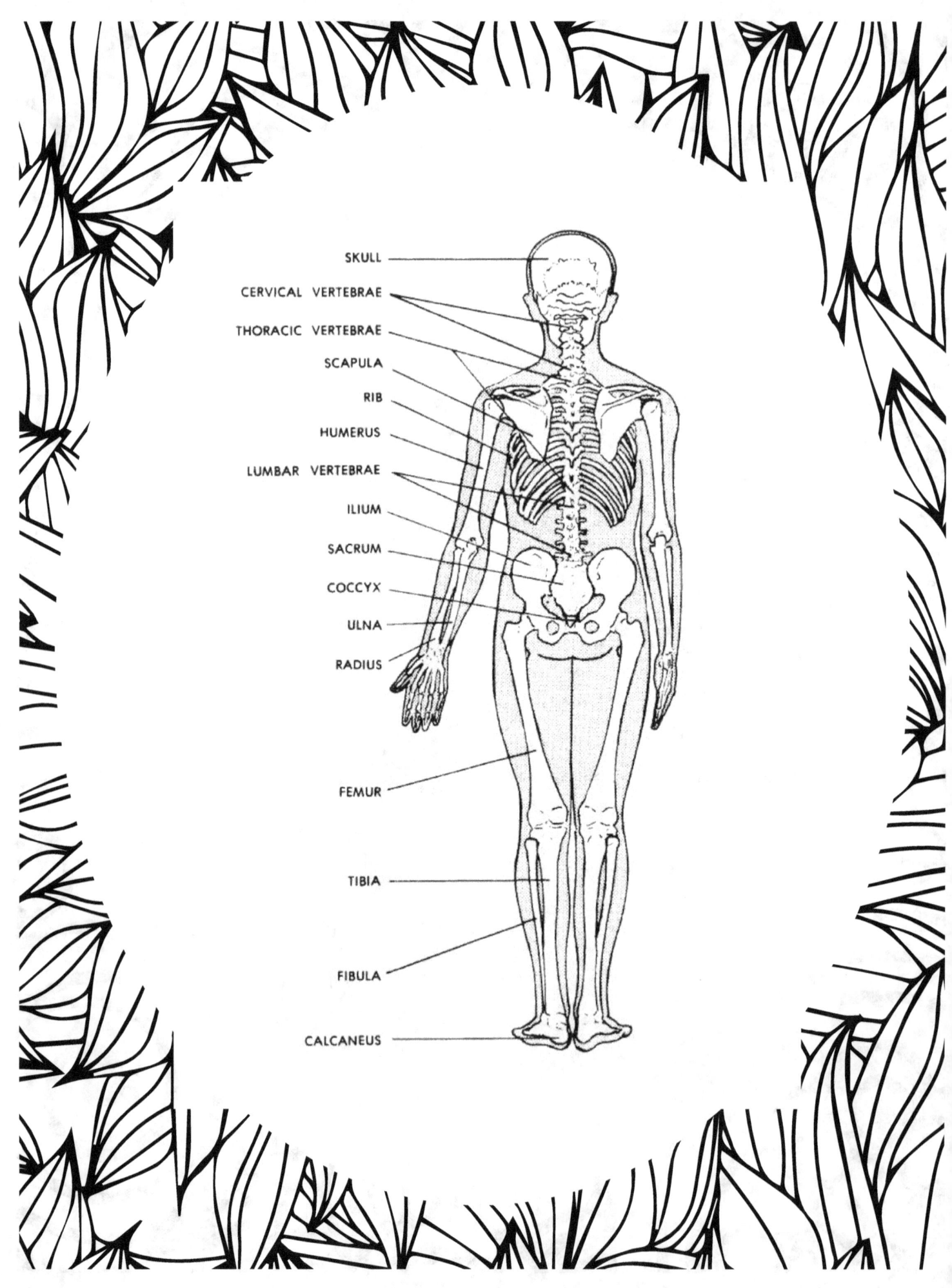

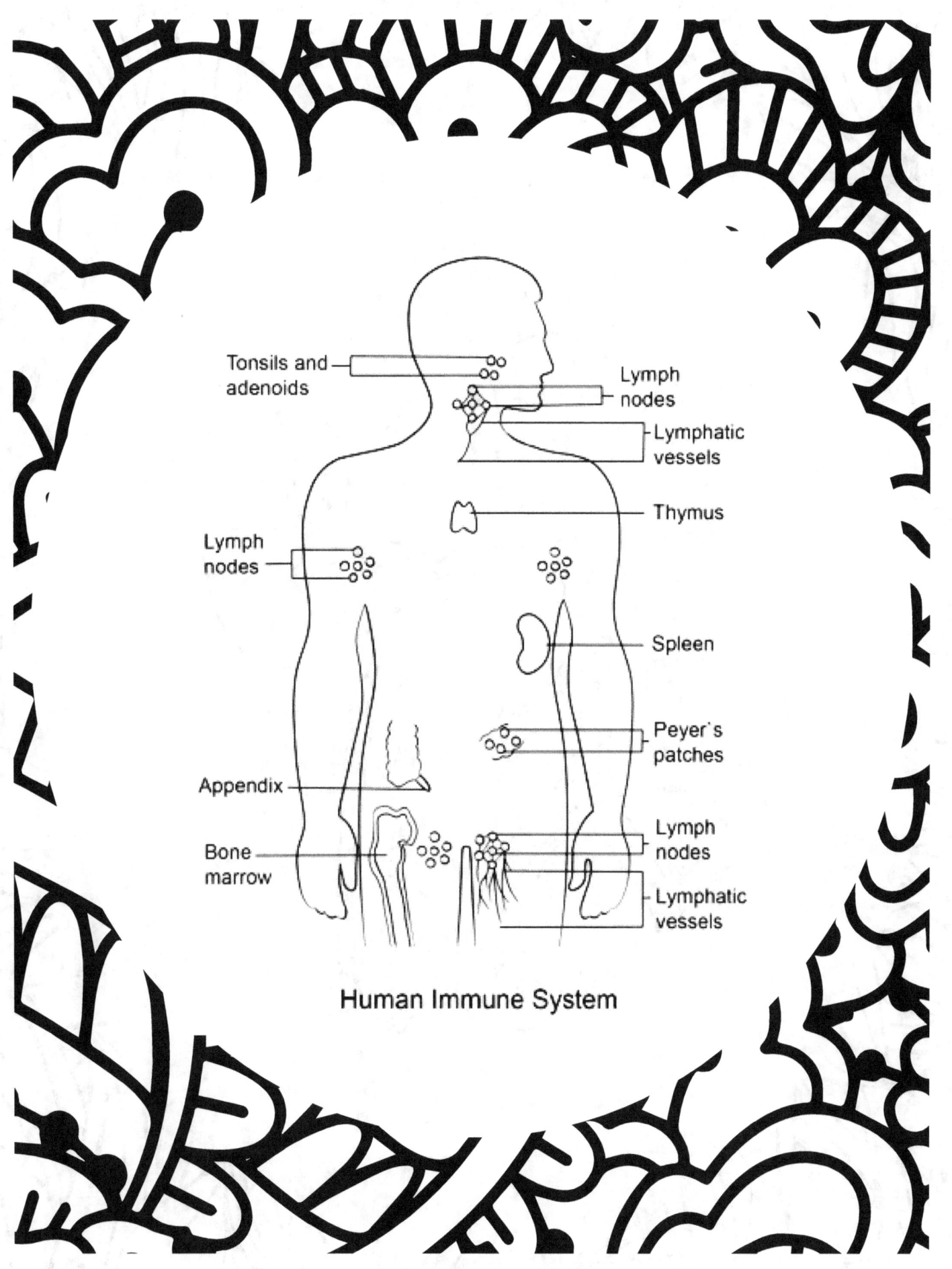

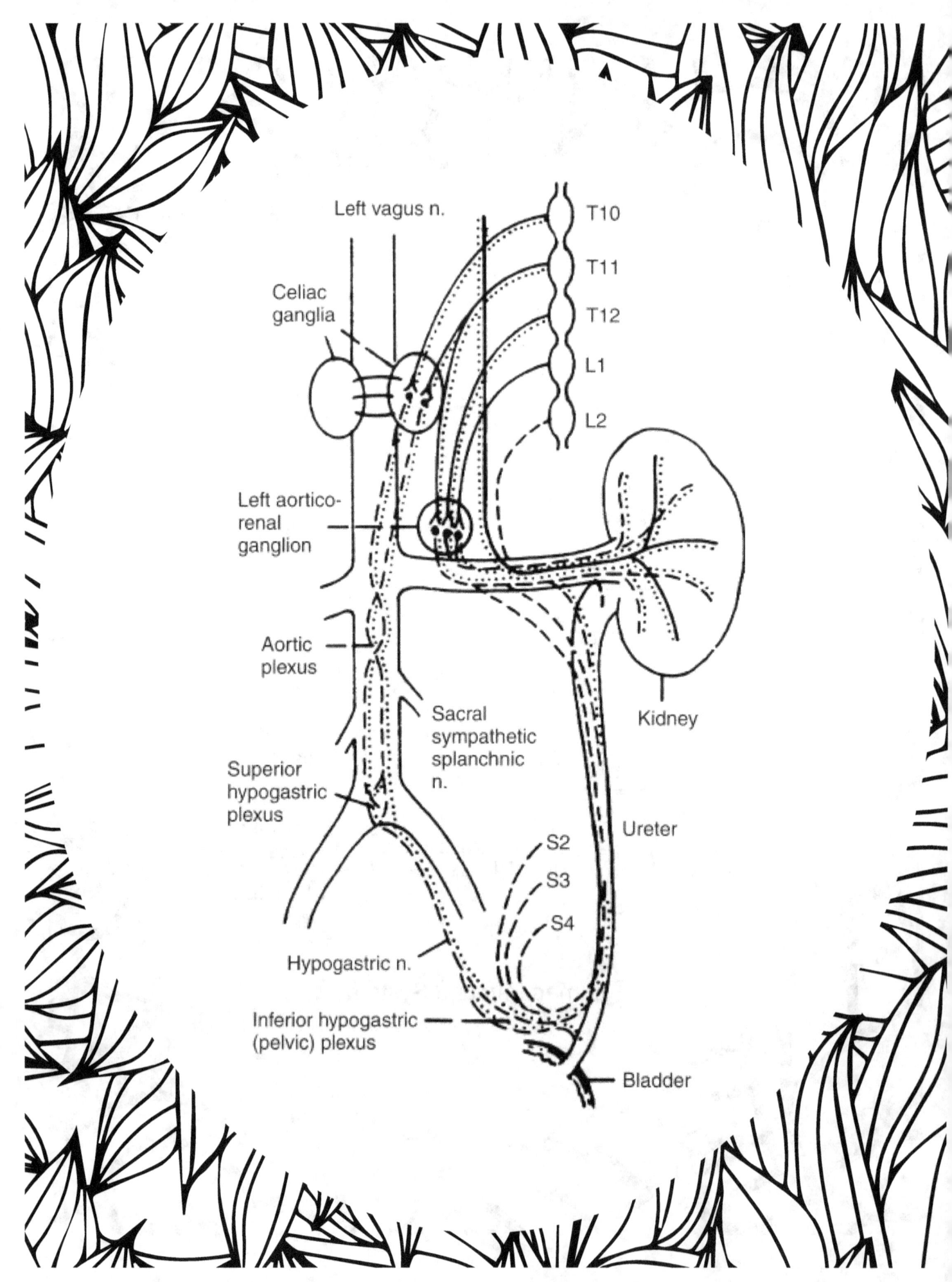

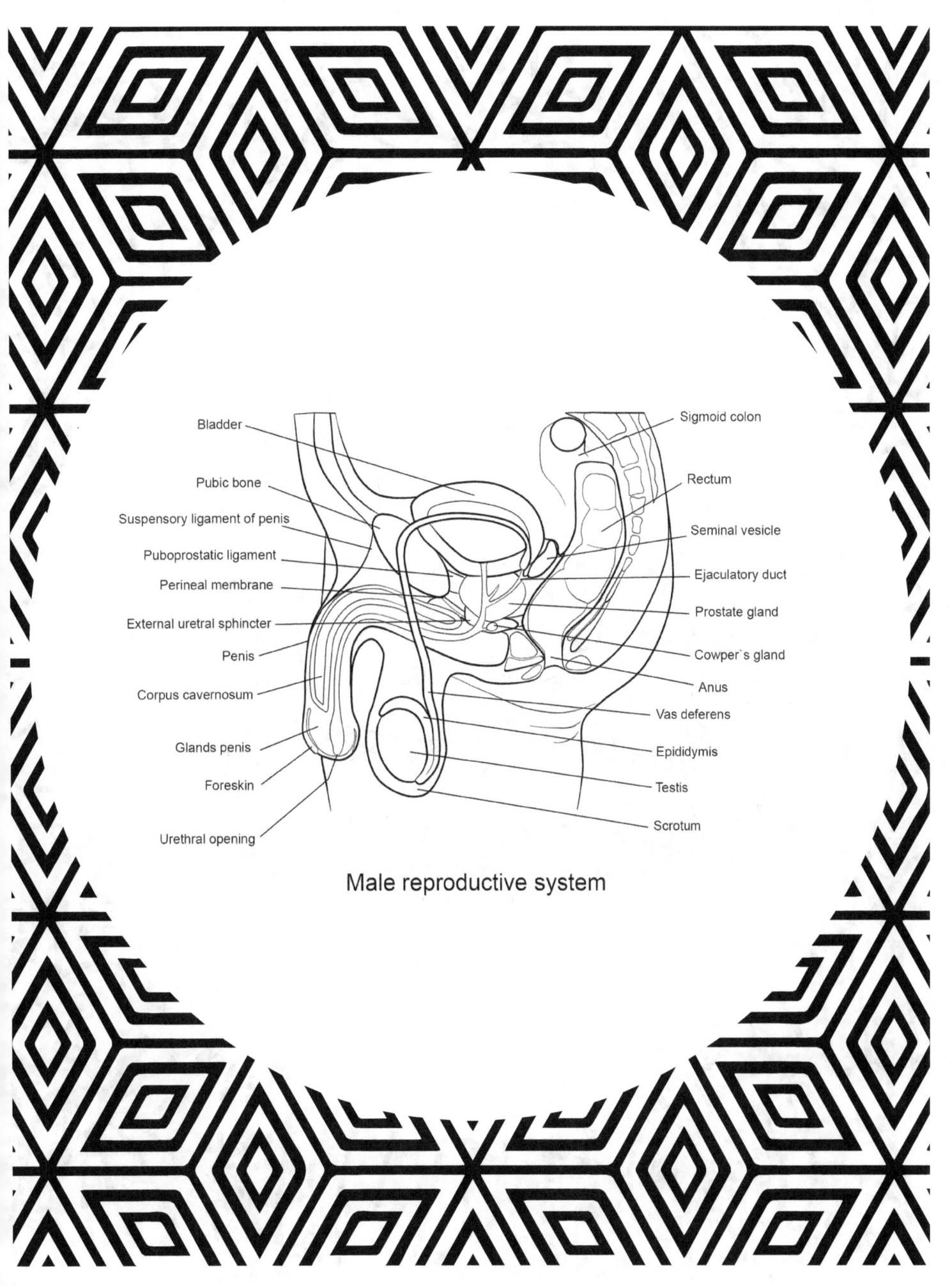

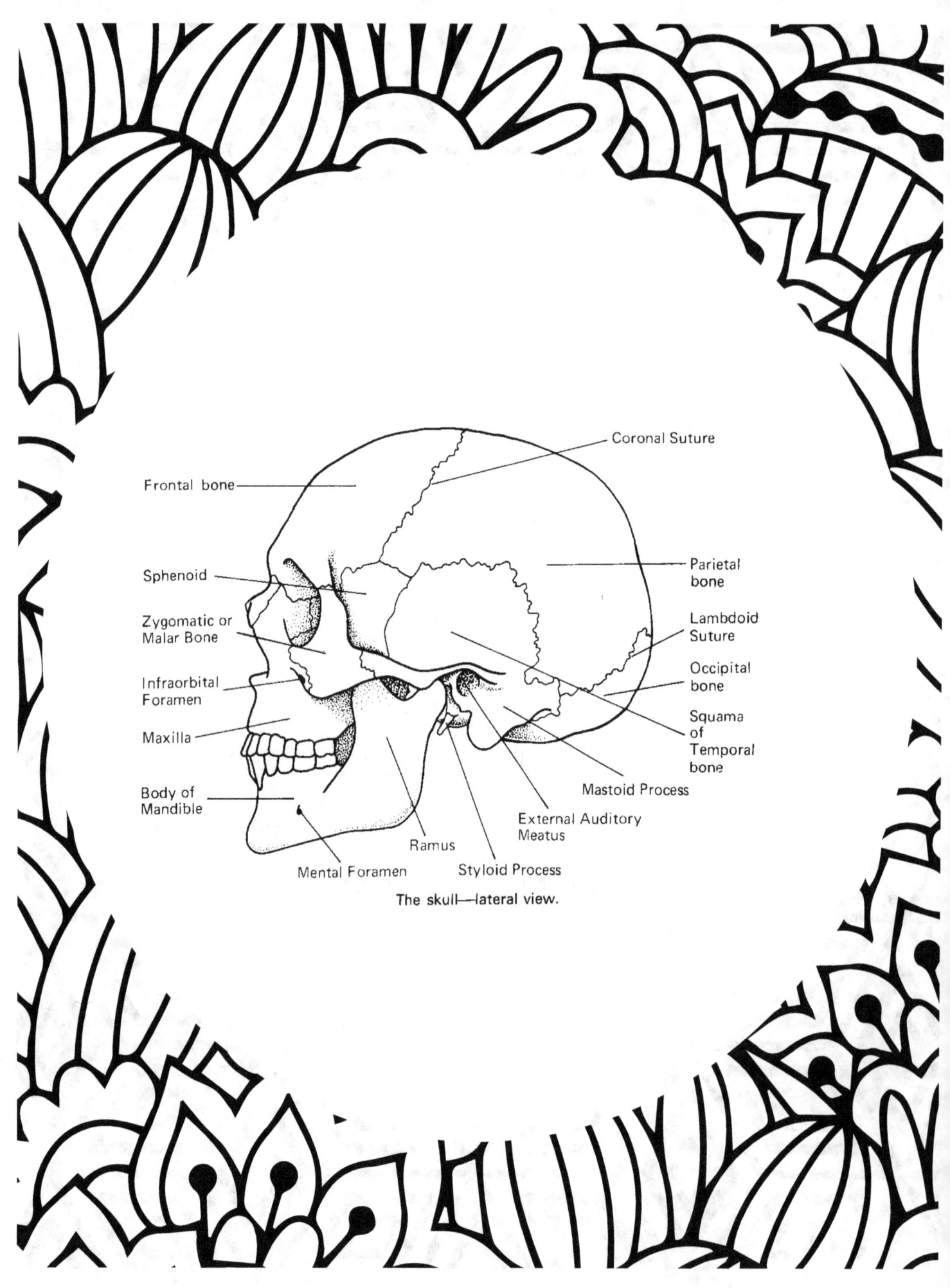

The skull—lateral view.

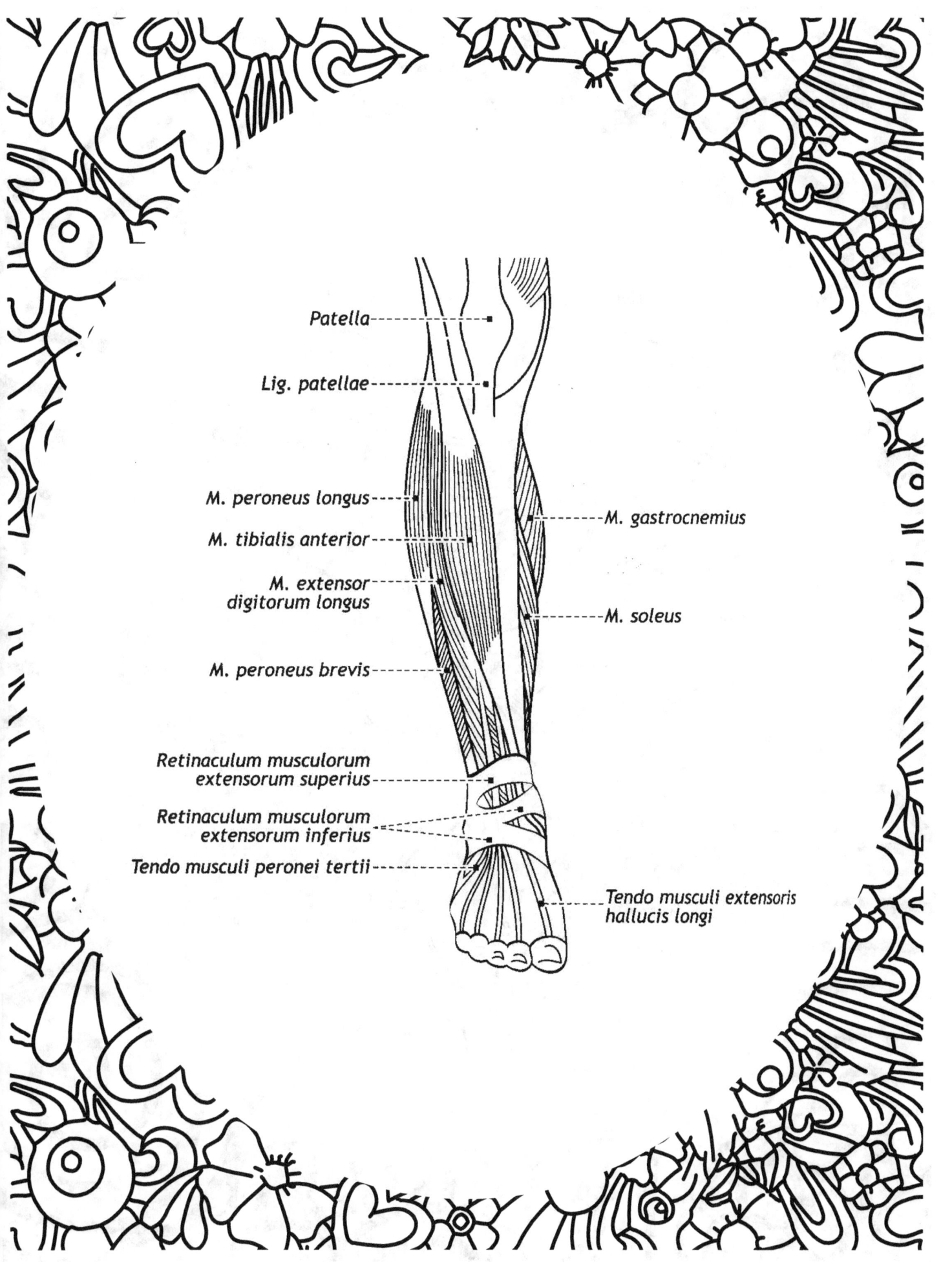

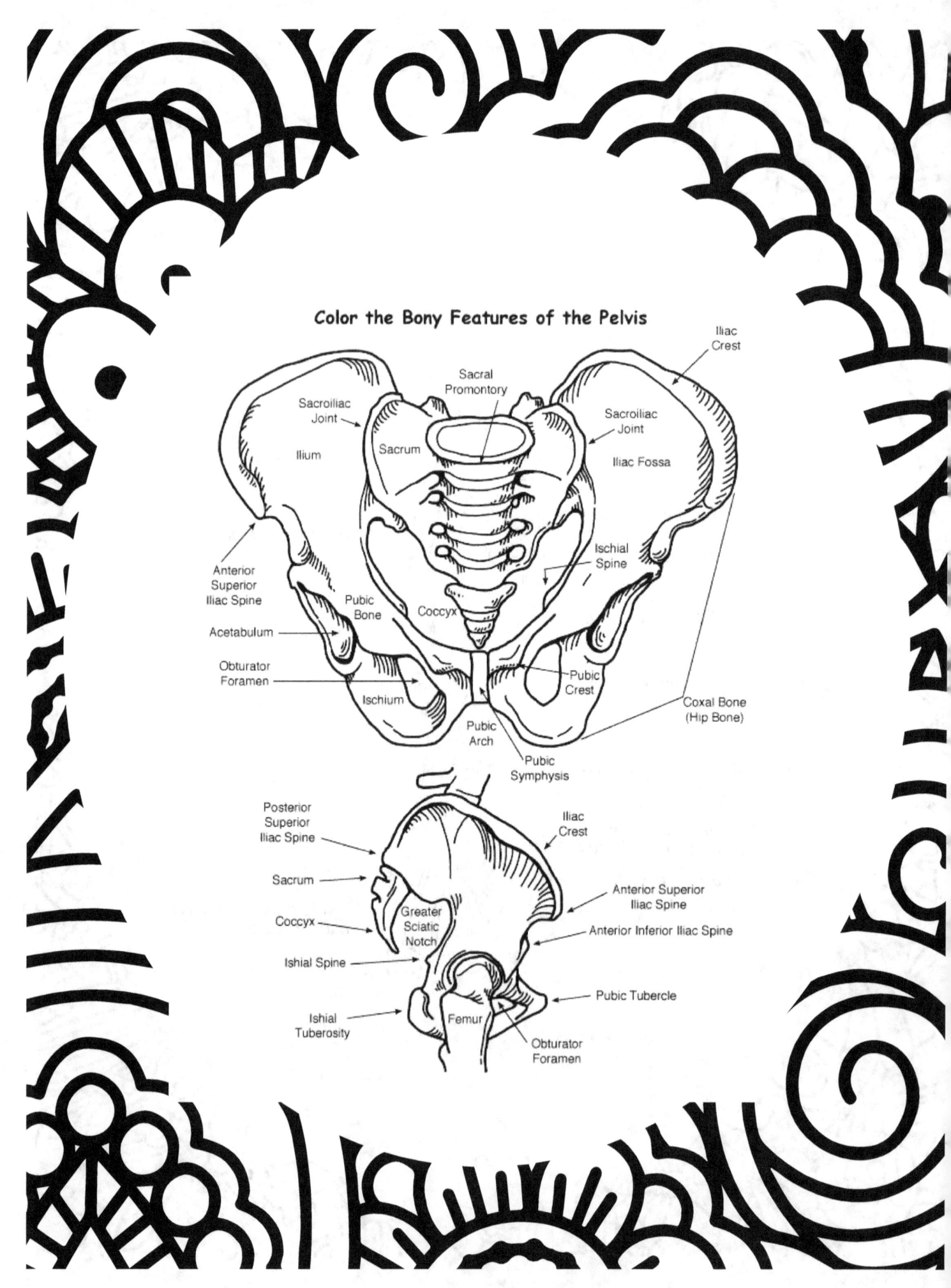

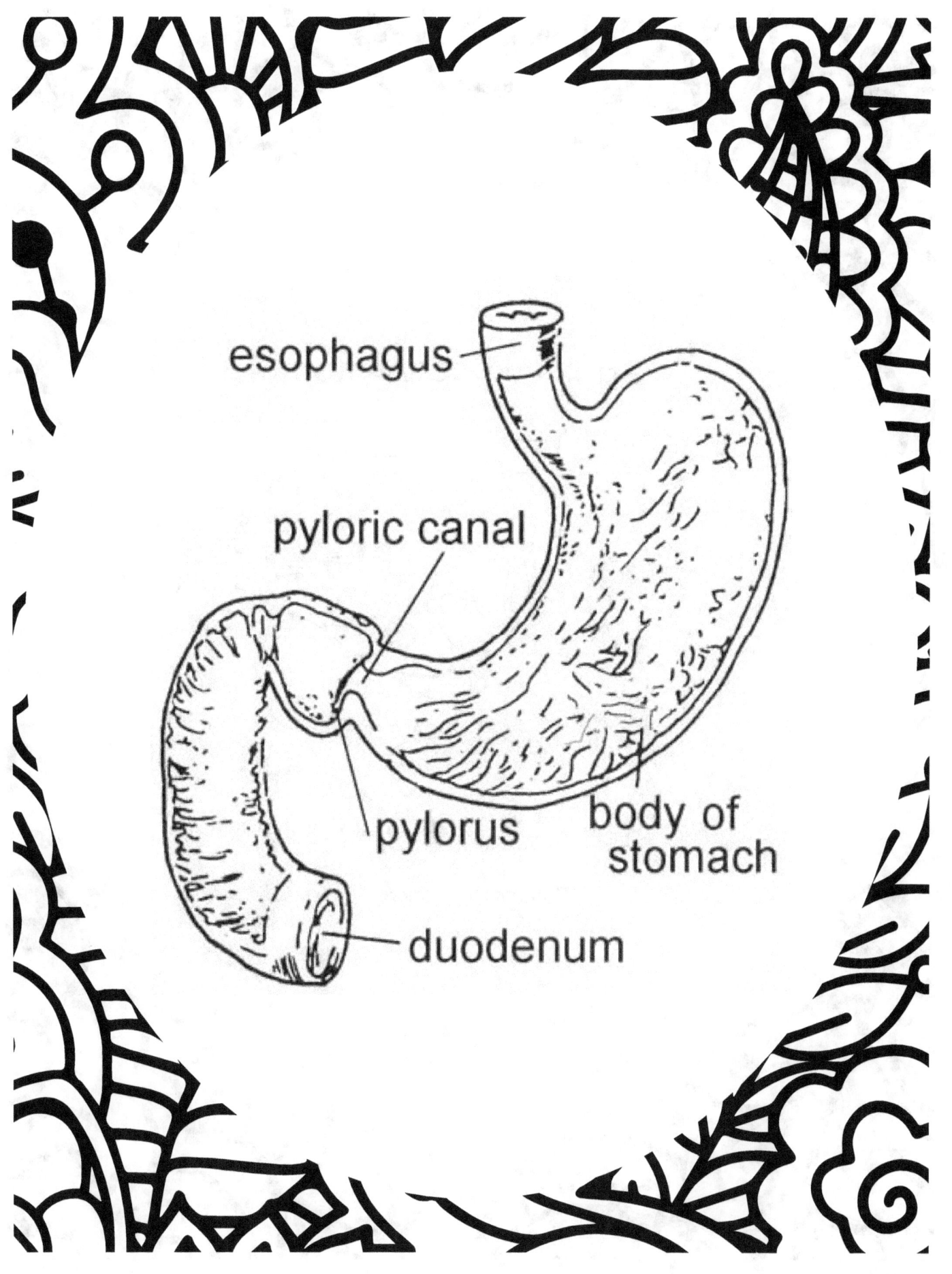

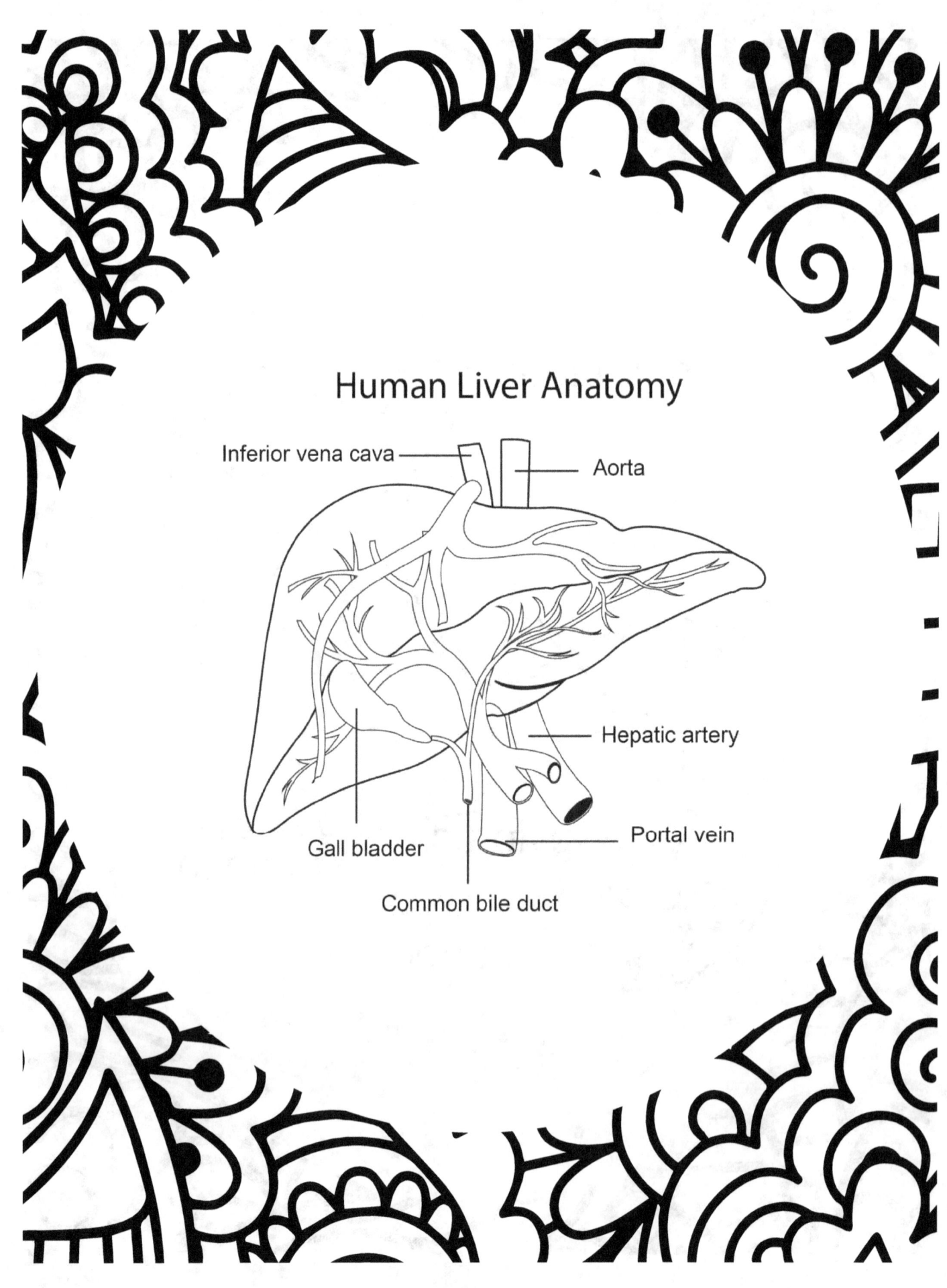

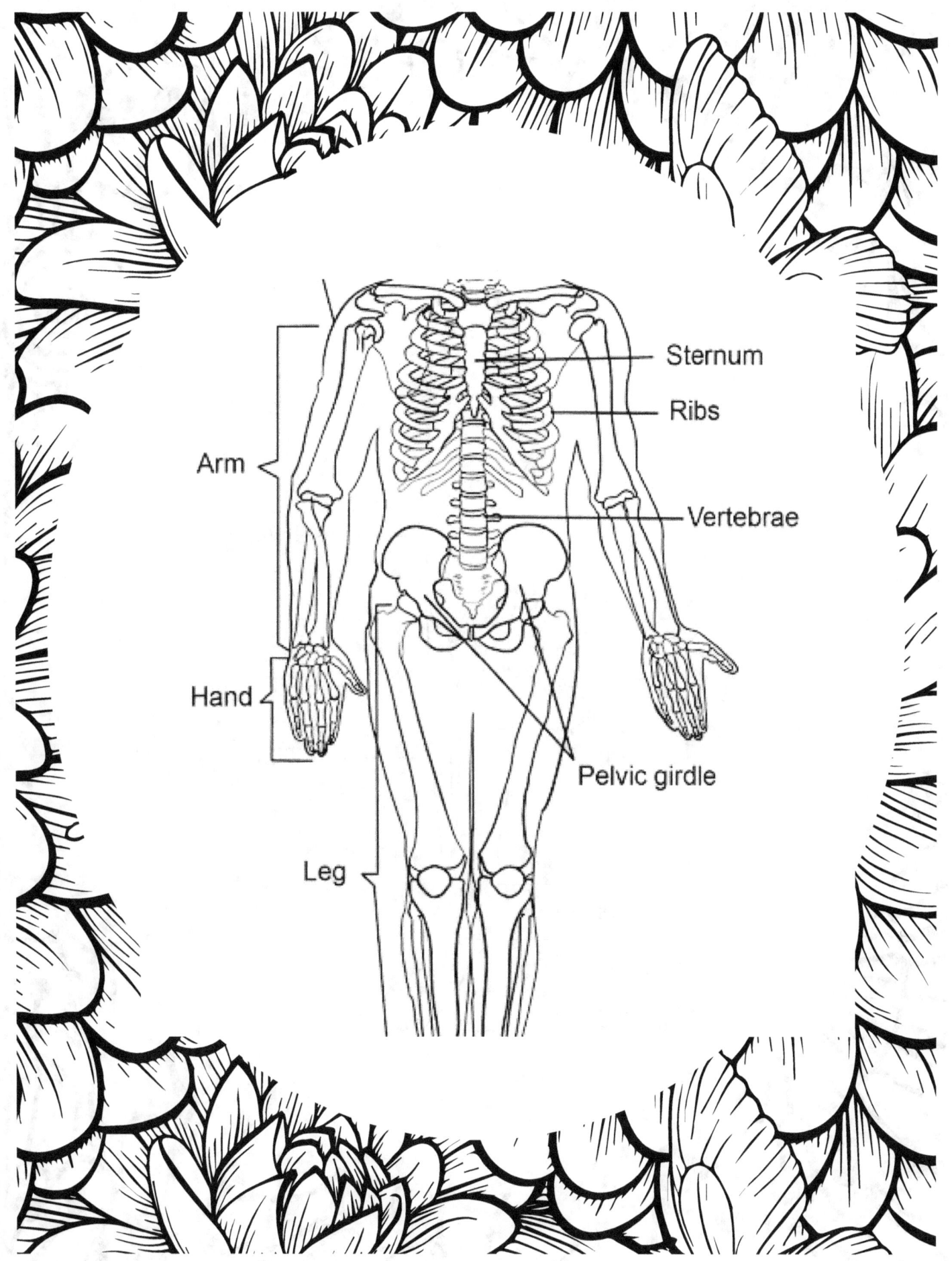

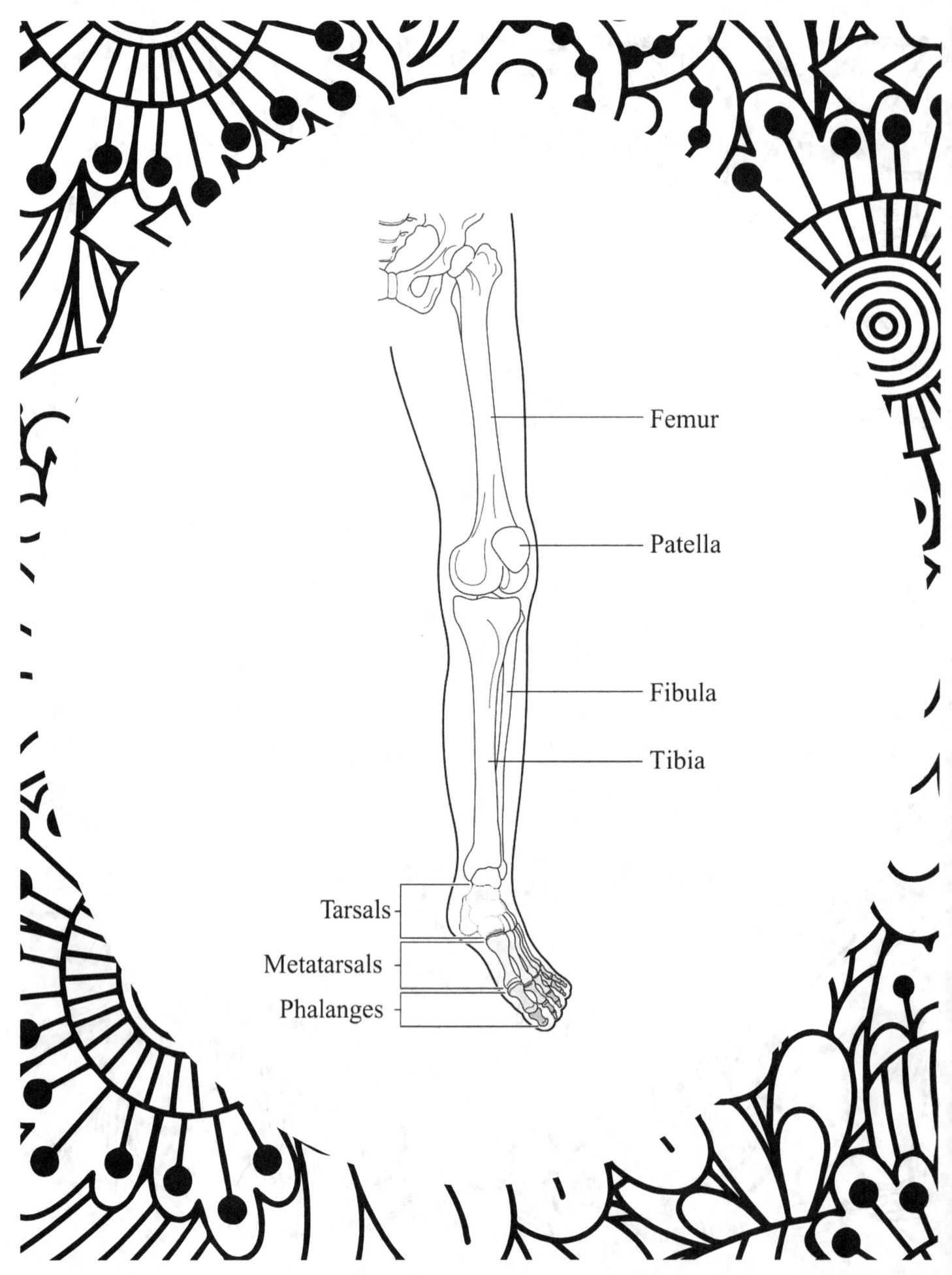

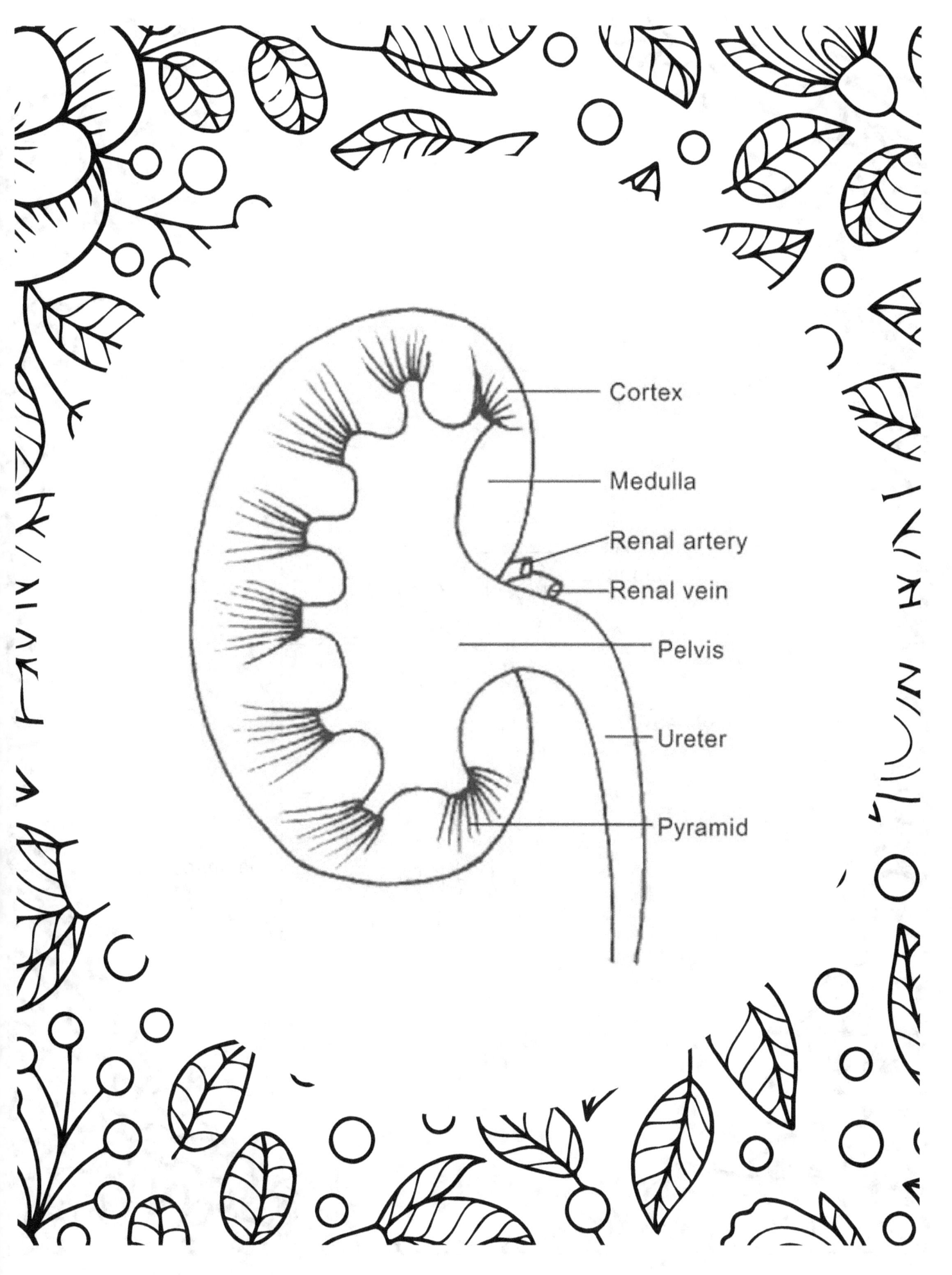

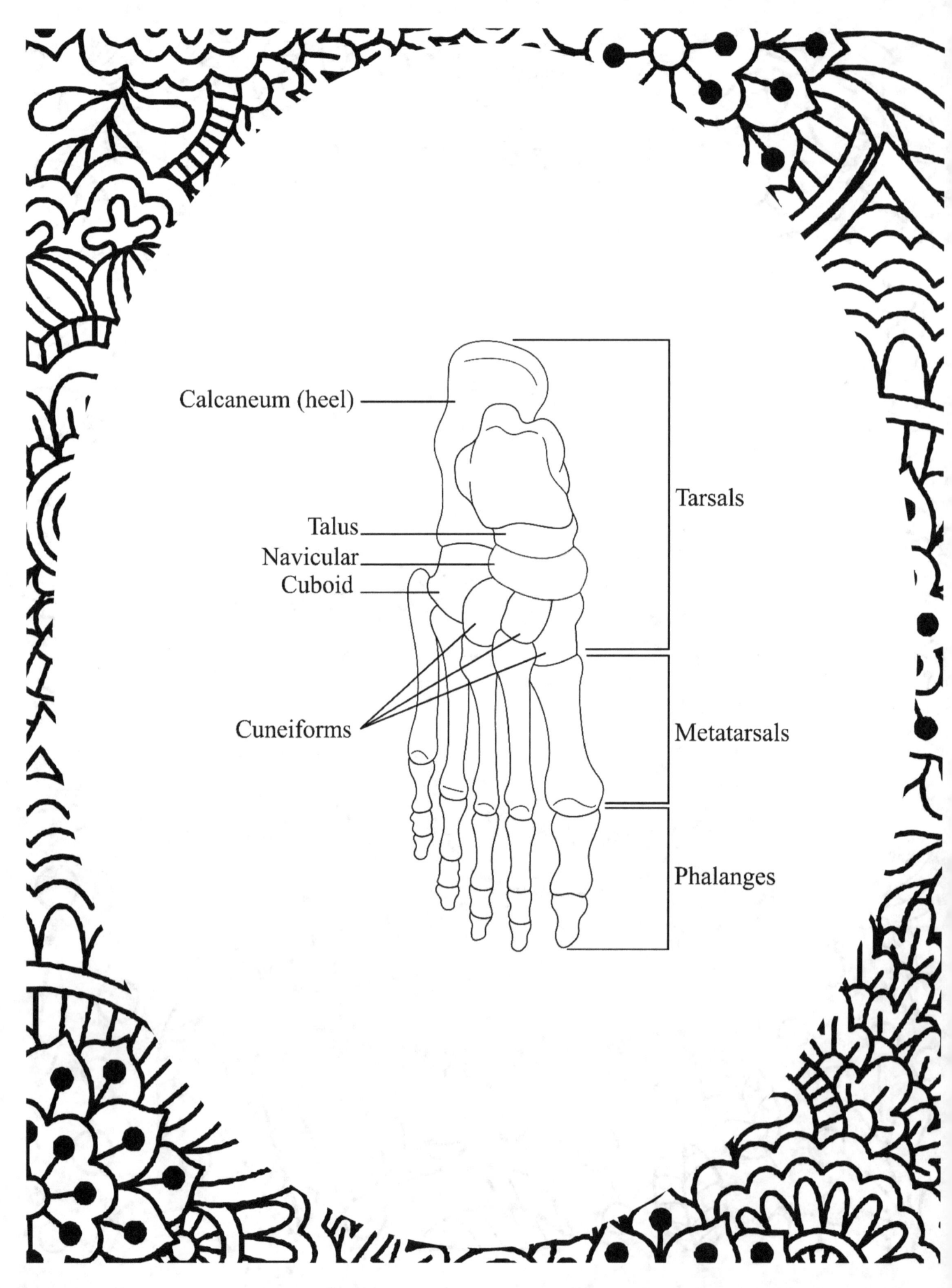

Color the Arteries of the Head and Neck

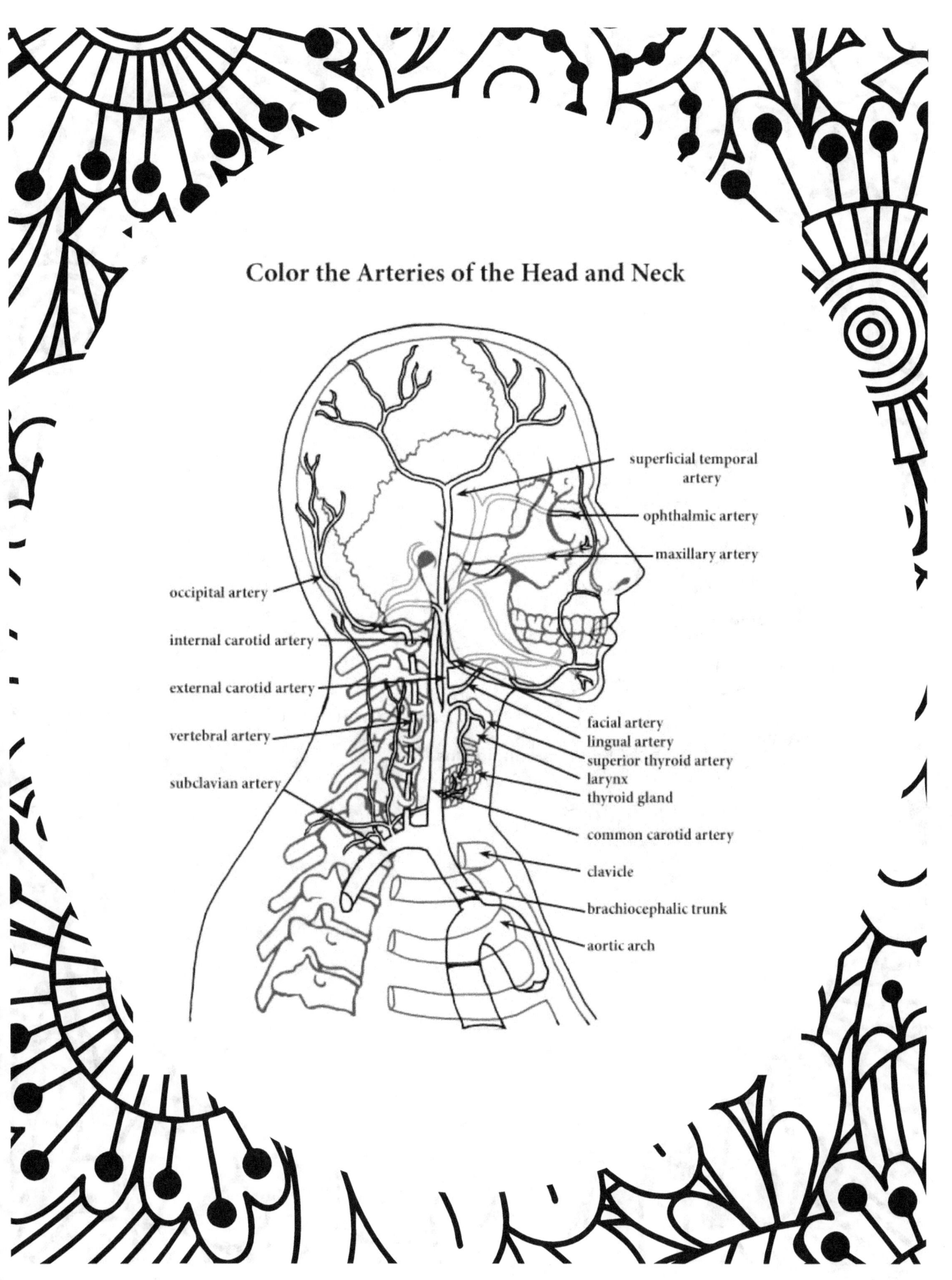

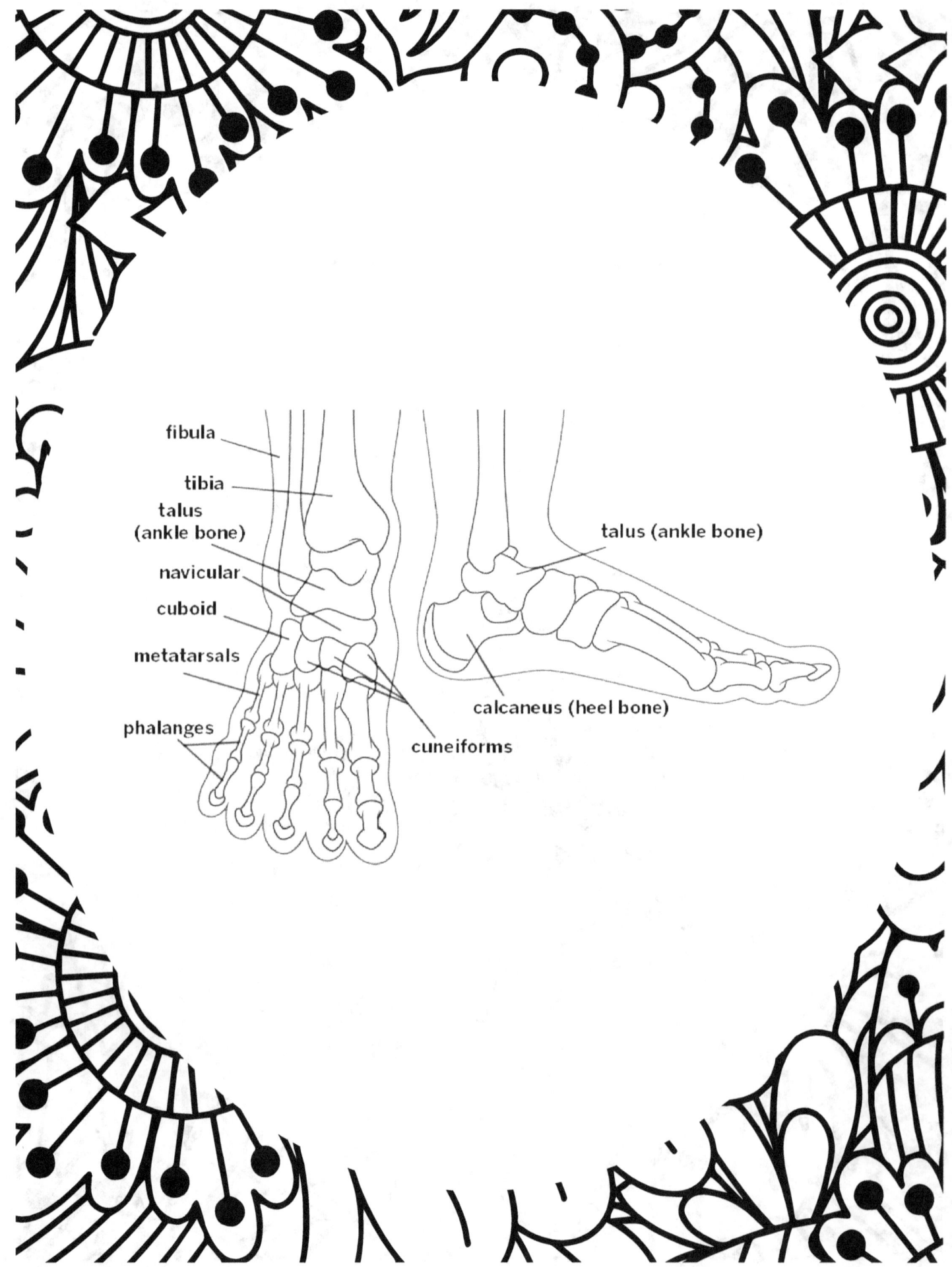

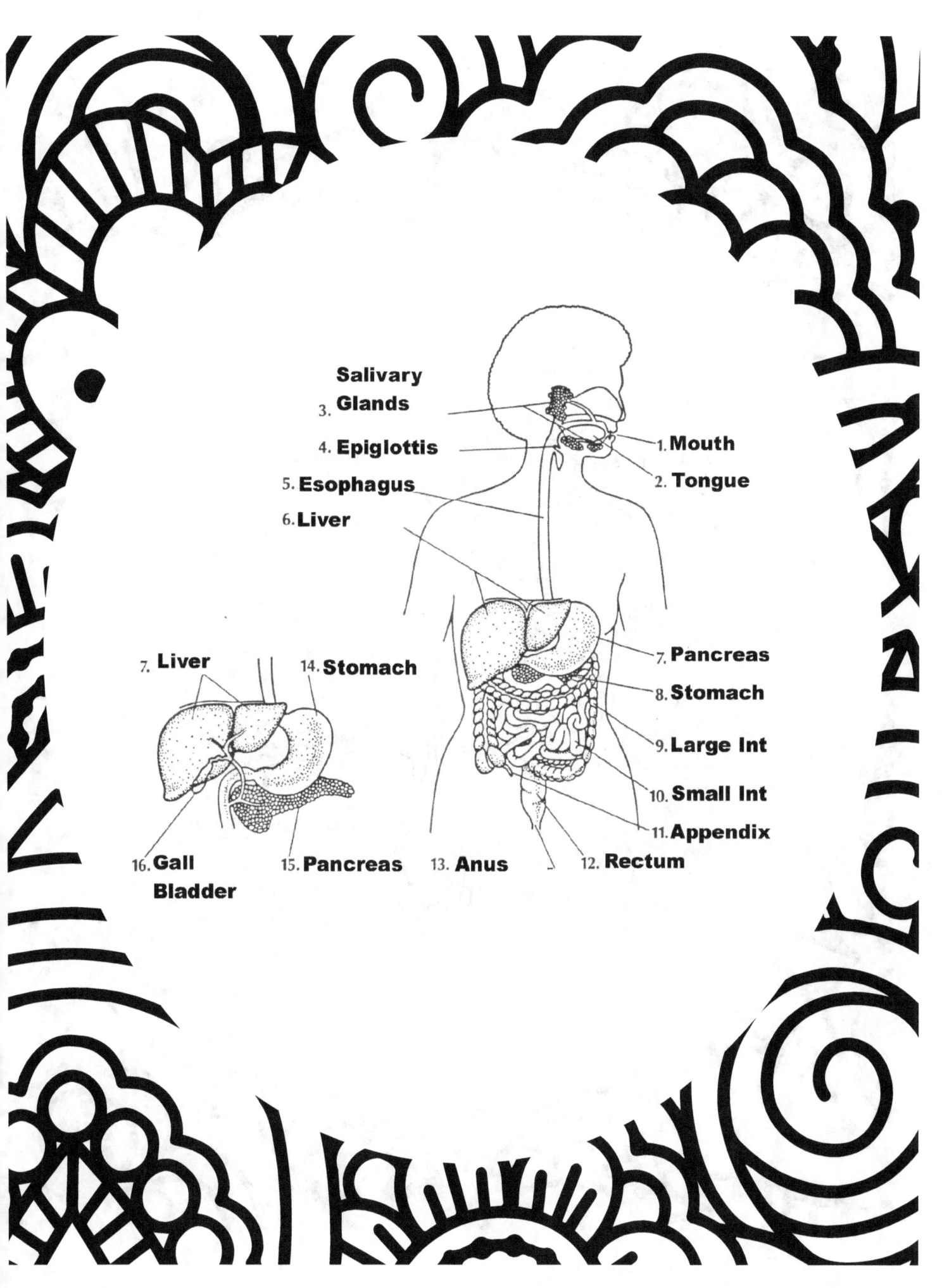

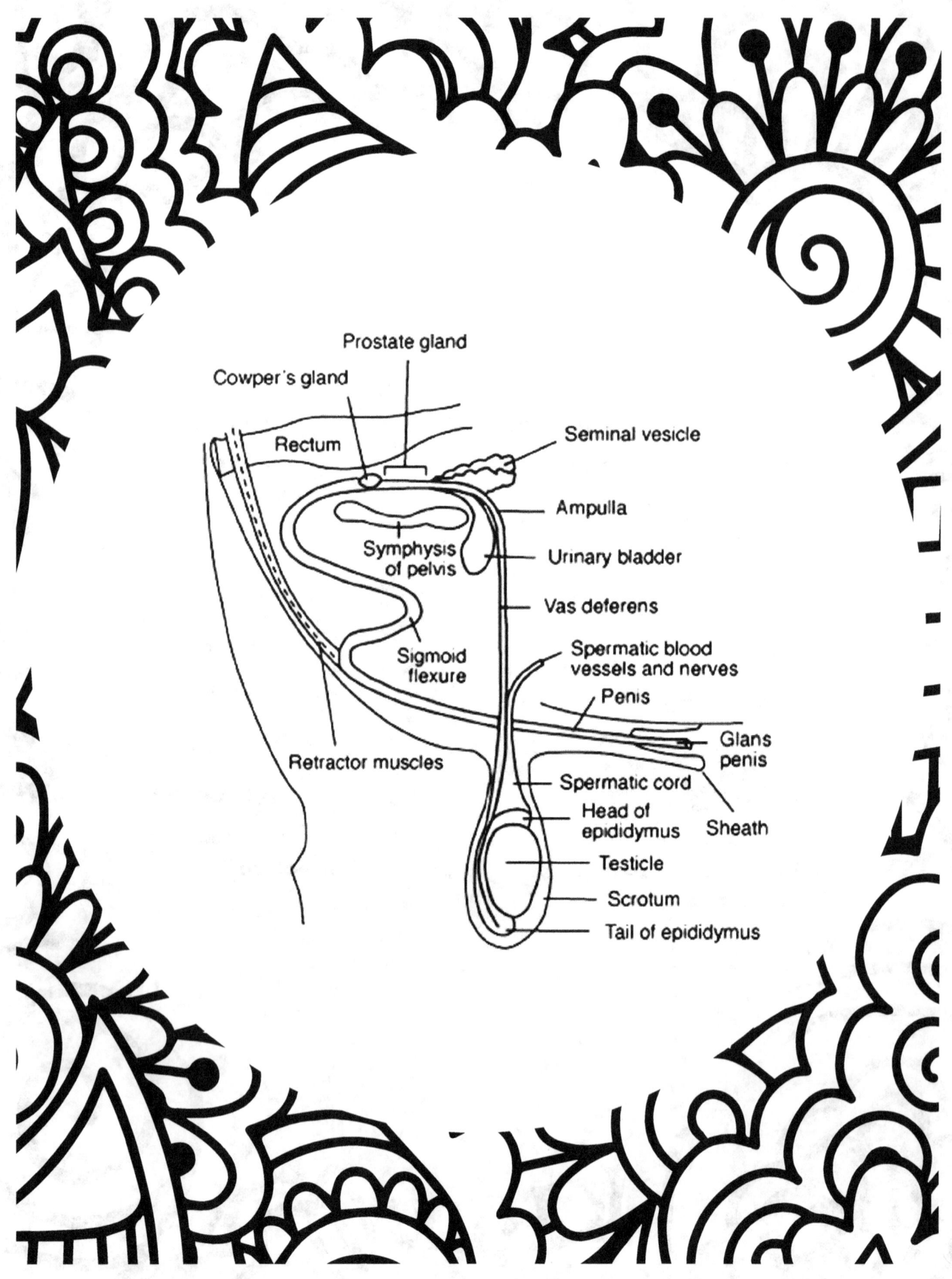

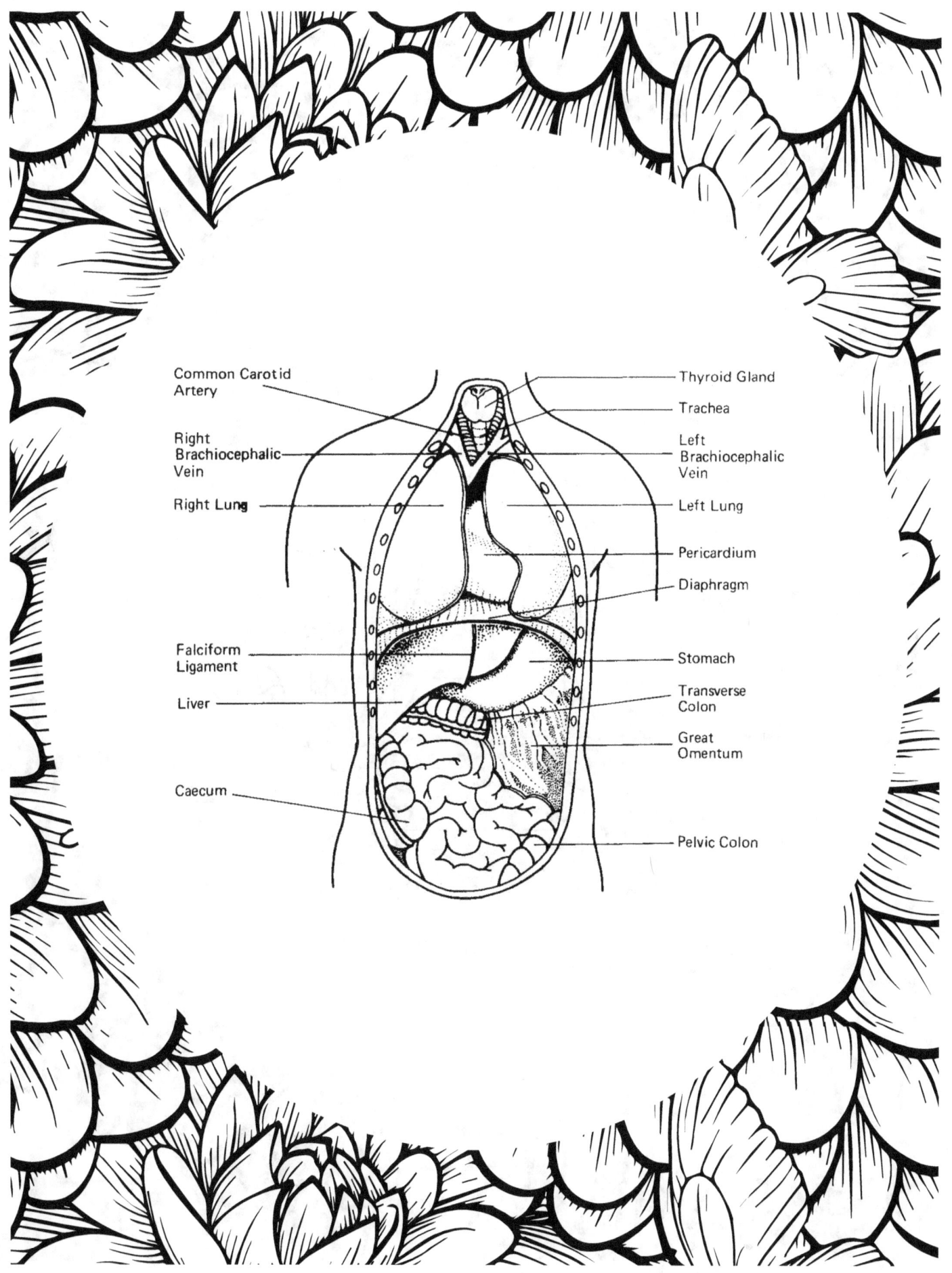

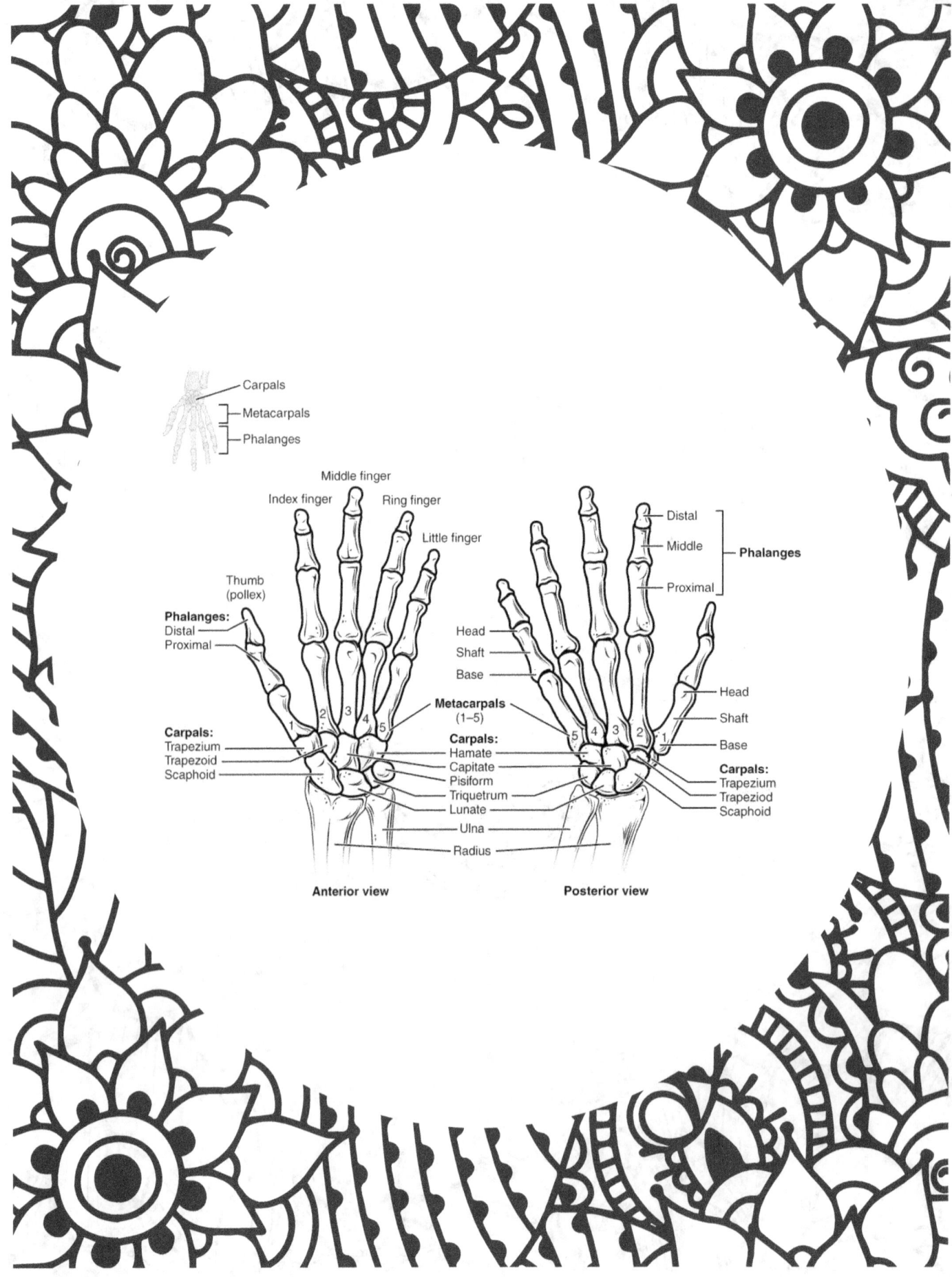

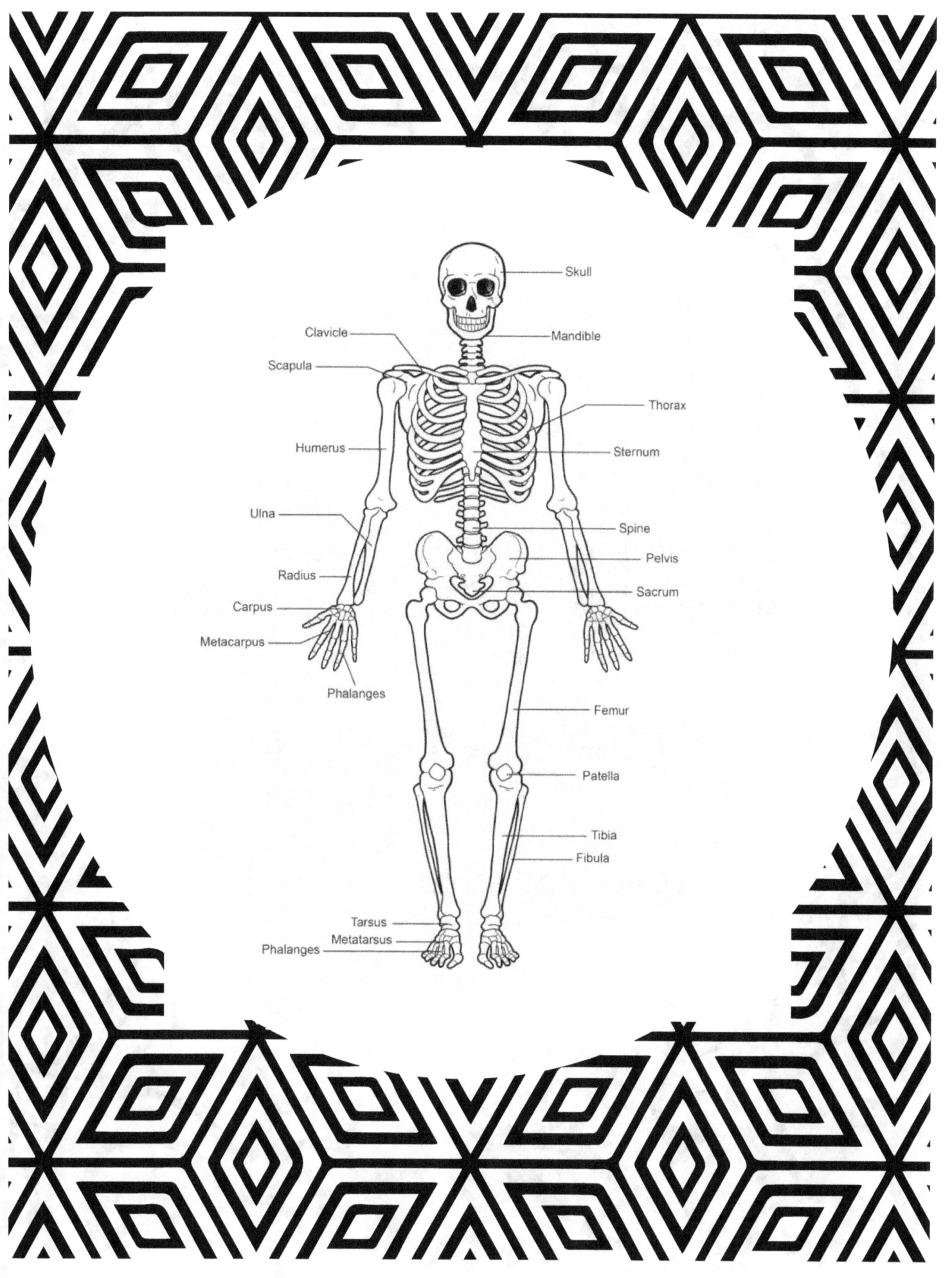

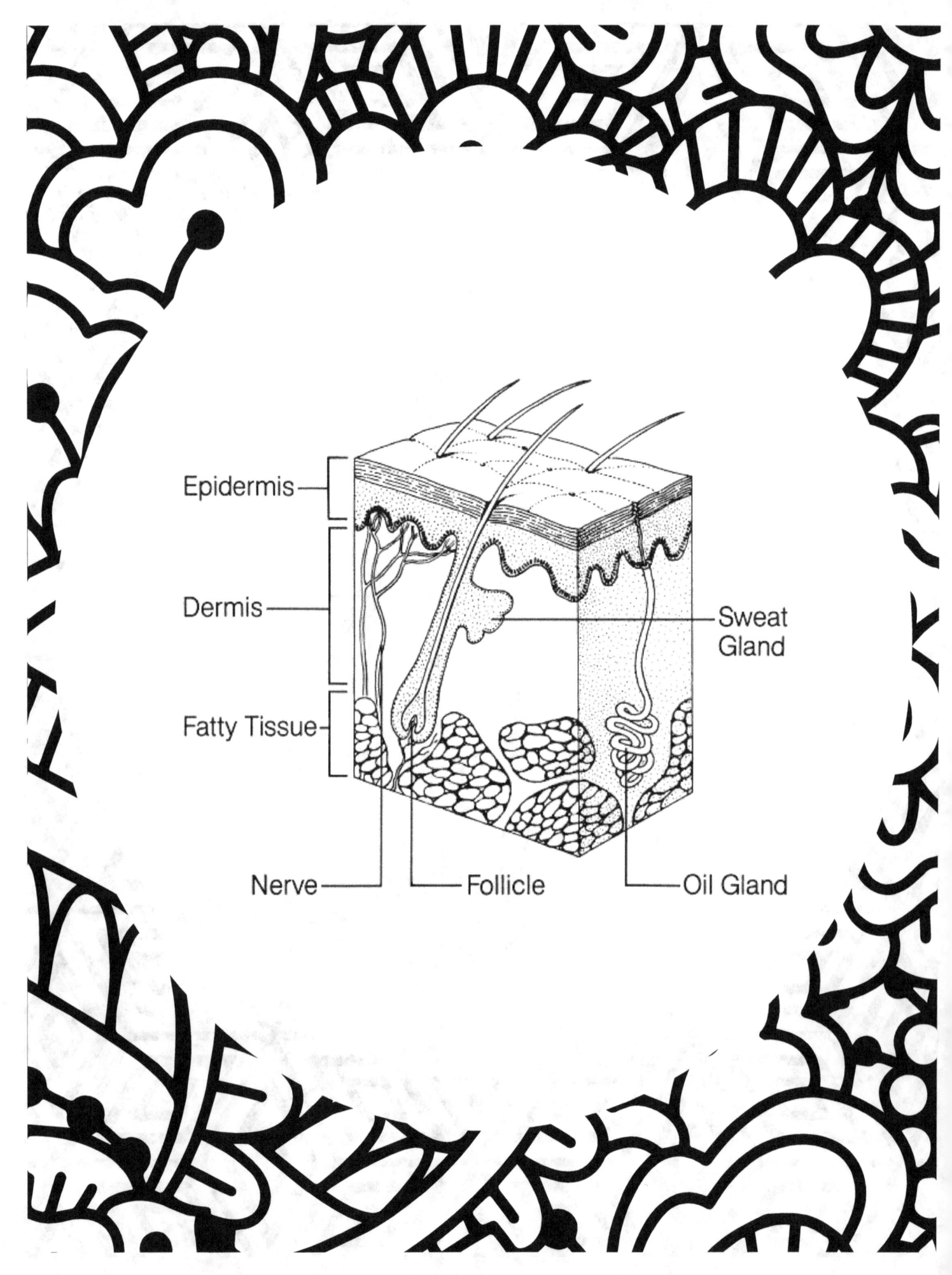

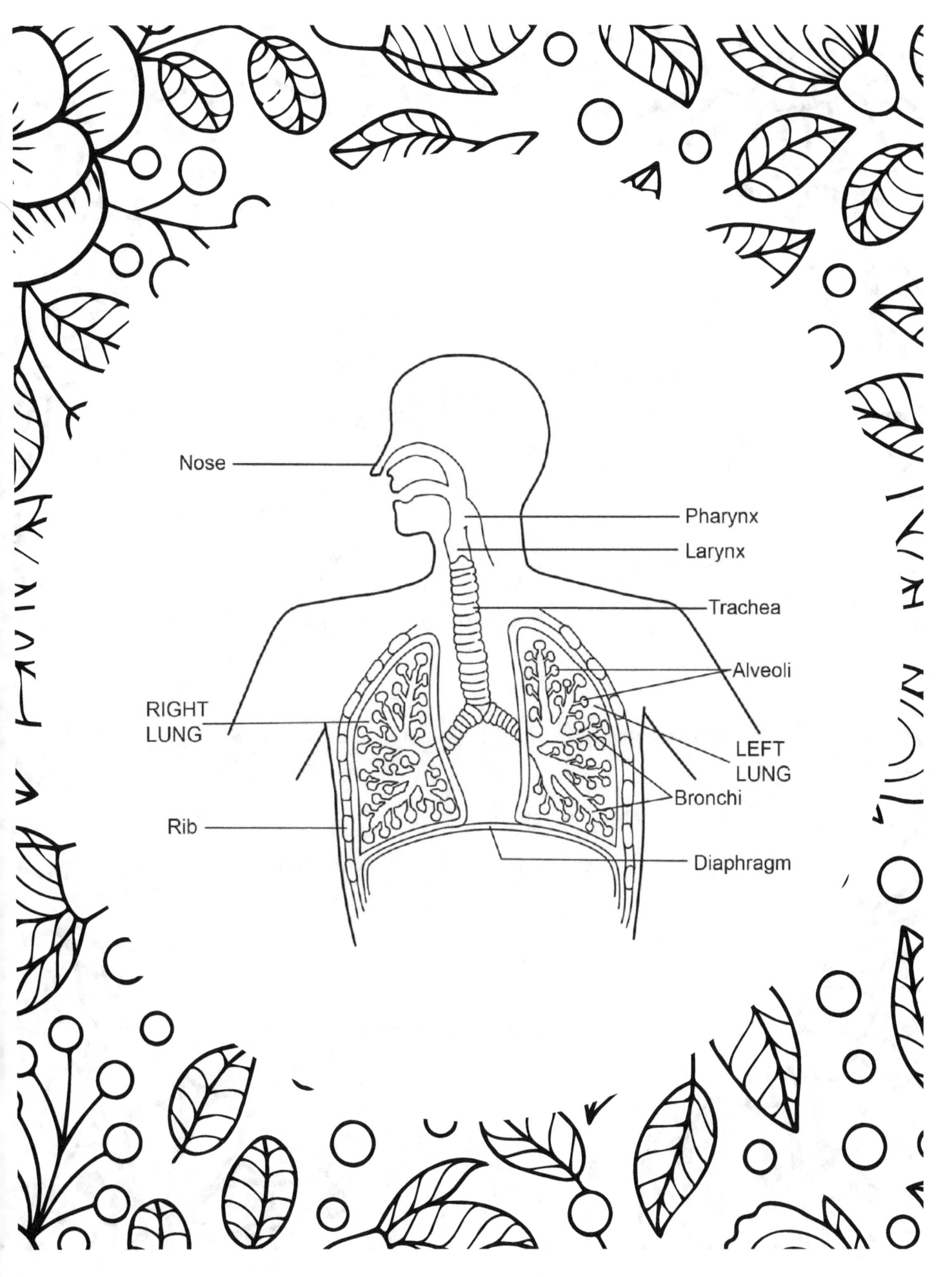

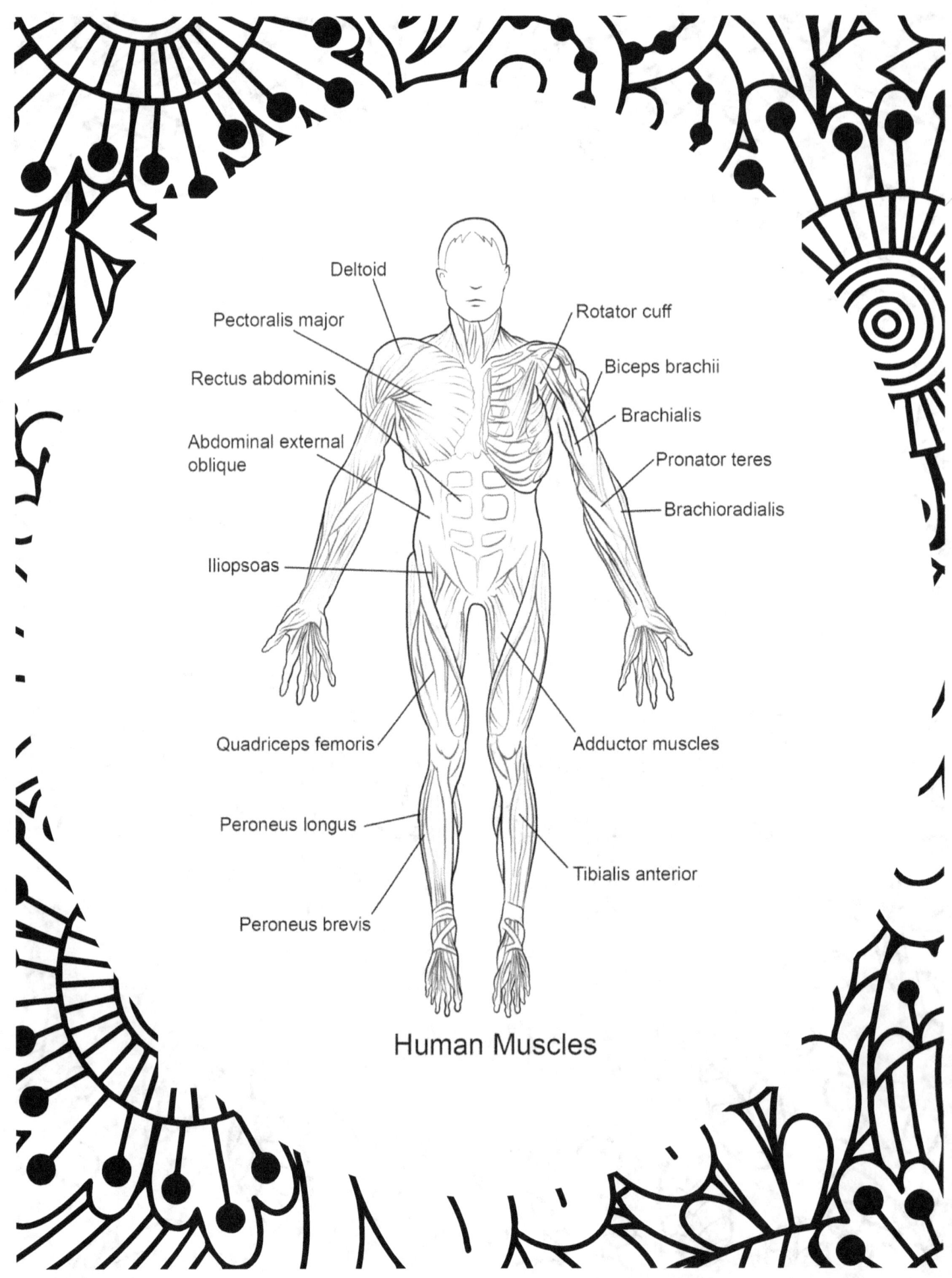

www.ingramcontent.com/pod-product-compliance
Lightning Source LLC
Chambersburg PA
CBHW081700220526

45466CB00009B/2839